Transcending Aging

♦

Stay Young Through the Power of Your Beliefs

Anet Paulina

iUniverse, Inc.
New York Lincoln Shanghai

Transcend the Aging Process
Stay Young Through the Power of Your Beliefs

All Rights Reserved © 2004 by Anet Paulina

No part of this book may be reproduced or transmitted in any form or by any means, graphic, electronic, or mechanical, including photocopying, recording, taping, or by any information storage retrieval system, without the written permission of the publisher.

iUniverse, Inc.

For information address:
iUniverse, Inc.
2021 Pine Lake Road, Suite 100
Lincoln, NE 68512
www.iuniverse.com

The author of this book does not dispense medical advice or prescribe the use of any treatment for physical or psychological problems. The intent of the author is only to offer information of a general nature to help you in your quest for personal growth. In the event that you use any of the information in this book for yourself, the author and publisher assume no responsibility for your actions.

ISBN: 0-595-31812-6

Printed in the United States of America

Contents

Introduction 1

Part I Paradigm Shift

Chapter 1 The New View of Aging 7
Old Ideas About Aging 7
A New Paradigm 10
The Biology of Belief 13
Your Body Reflects Your Beliefs 15
Why Does Aging Occur? 18

Chapter 2 Limiting Beliefs About Aging 19
Consciousness Shift 19
Beliefs and Truths 19
You Control Your Body 20
Models of Youthfulness 22
Celebrating Birthdays 23
Realigning "Old" Beliefs 25

Part II Mind Matters

Chapter 3 Developing Awareness 31
Paying Attention 31
Thought, Emotion, and Intuition 32
Meditation 34
Breathing 36
Challenges to Awareness 38

Chapter 4 Conscious Creation 41
Creating Our Own Reality 41
Energy Follows Attention 42
How Creation Works 43
Impediments to Creation.................................. 45
Creating Wealth 51
Body Consciousness...................................... 53

Chapter 5 Emotional Clearing 57
Self-Acceptance 57
Judgment and Negativity.................................. 59
Attaining Acceptance..................................... 60
Clearing the Past 63
Energy Psychology....................................... 66

Part III *Physical Strategies*

Chapter 6 Health Without Hype 73
Health Responsibility..................................... 73
Health Care Services 74
Why Treatments Don't Work 78
Why Health Problems Occur.............................. 79
Energy Healing 81
A Healthy Environment................................... 83

Chapter 7 Nutrition Without a Diet Plan. 87
What (and When) to Eat.................................. 87
Special Dietary Concerns.................................. 89
Nutritional Sources 91
Herbalism 95
Wonderful Water... 96
Weight Management 97

Chapter 8 Fitness Without a Regimen 99
Don't Act Your Age....................................... 99
Develop an Exercise Habit................................. 100

    Use Your "Other" Hand 101
    The Tibetan Rites of Rejuvenation 102
    The Energy Centers 105

CHAPTER 9   Personal Care Without a Product Line 111
    Skin Care 111
    Sun Exposure 113
    Hair Care 116
    Dental Care 116
    Vision Care 117
    Plastic Surgery 118

Part IV   *Additional Areas*

CHAPTER 10   Streamlining and Simplifying 123
    Old Stuff Leads to Old Folks 123
    Streamlining Suggestions 124
    Use It or Lose It 125
    Managing New Purchases 127
    Your Stuff and Your Identity 128

CHAPTER 11   The Ultimate Taboo 129
    The Longevity Question 129
    An Alternative View of Death 130
    The Mystery of Life After Death 131
    Continuing Communication 132
    A Broader Perspective 134

Afterword 137

Notes 139

Resources 143

Glossary 147

Index 155

Acknowledgements

To John Mekis, thank you for acting as a sounding board as these ideas were developed, reviewing the manuscript, taking the author photograph, providing computer support, and—most of all—for having faith in me.

To Dr. Bruce Lipton, thank you for offering encouragement and allowing me to use your material.

For presenting information that helped broaden my awareness and shift my perspective in fundamental ways, I thank Seth, Jane Roberts, and Rob Butts for the Seth material; and Elias, Mary Ennis, Vicki Pendley, Paul and Joanne Helfrich, Bobbi Houle, and all others who have helped make the Elias material available to the public. Mary, thank you for allowing me to use the Elias material on energy centers.

For reviewing the manuscript and providing helpful suggestions and encouragement, I thank Edward Vajda, Paul Tews, and Kevin Aho.

To Marcy, Barbara, and others who shared their views and experiences with me, I offer a heartfelt "thank you."

Without the contributions of these people (and probably some others I may have unintentionally left out), this book would not exist in its present form.

Introduction

Here's the billion-dollar question: What is the secret to staying youthful regardless of chronological age? Is it even possible?

The answer is yes—it is possible. Whether it is possible for *you* depends upon whether or not you believe it's possible. The key to lifelong youth is simply believing—truly knowing—that the way you experience aging is completely up to you. As with many things in life, simple isn't necessarily easy.

To those who may ask, "What's wrong with aging?" the answer is that there is nothing wrong with getting older, nor is age-related degeneration inherently bad. The manner in which we age is neither bad not good; it's simply a choice of experience. If you are reading this book, then I assume your preference is to remain youthful as you get older, so I'm approaching the subject from that perspective.

I would like to make it clear from the start that I'm not a medical professional and have no advanced degrees or certifications, nor do I claim to be an authority on health or anti-aging. (The term *anti-aging* makes me cringe, but I haven't come up with a more positive yet succinct way to describe the avoidance of age-related degeneration.) If that's what you're looking for, there certainly is no dearth of professionals with a string of letters behind their names who say they have solutions to the problems attributed to aging. My approach is much broader in perspective, as well as somewhat unconventional. It includes making use of findings about the rejuvenating effects of nutrition and other practices, but the core idea is to fundamentally alter the way we perceive aging.

My "credentials" are a lifelong interest and over 30 years of study in health, fitness, nutrition, psychology, personal growth, and metaphysics, which led me to seek out information about the keys for staying youthful throughout life. My interest in psychoneuroimmunology (the study of how the mind affects the body) was sparked in the early 1980s when I read a newspaper article about Dr. Candace Pert's discoveries on the biology of emotion. Mind-body interactions, energy healing, intuition, and psychic phenomena fascinated me for many years before they came into vogue.

At this point you may be wondering, "Why does this woman think she knows more about aging than scientists and doctors do?" I wouldn't put the question in quite those terms. I don't necessarily know more, but I *am* aware of some crucial factors that most anti-aging researchers remain oblivious to. Professionals with extensive medical or scientific training and certifications have a vested interest in limiting their ideas to the tenets of those belief systems. When faced with new information that fundamentally shifts the paradigm in one's area of expertise, it's natural to resist change—especially when you've incorporated those beliefs so deeply that they seem like unalterable truths. I'm fortunate to have the freedom to stretch the boundaries of currently accepted scientific dogma without jeopardizing my professional standing.

A few years ago I began making notes of some of my ideas, not with the intention of writing a book, but simply because I thought they might be useful at some point. As I watched the post-World War II generation in their increasingly desperate quest to maintain or recover their youthful functioning and appearance, I realized that many people could benefit from what I've learned. In an exercise I sometimes use to clarify my priorities, I asked myself what I would most want to accomplish in the next year if I found out I had only one year left to live. The result is the book you are holding.

I've tried to strike a balance by offering information that doesn't perpetuate limiting beliefs, yet aligns closely enough with commonly held views that it will be of practical value to most readers. Keep in mind that the health-related information I'm presenting is based upon beliefs—as is all such information, regardless of the source. The suggestions I offer regarding heath, nutrition, fitness, and personal care are only tools; none of them is truly necessary for maintaining or regaining youthful functioning of the body and brain. They are methods that work within our present belief systems to make desired physical changes, which can strengthen our belief that we have control over the aging process.

Something I have purposely not done in this book is to provide scientific validation (study results or authorities cited) for all of the information included. I opted for this approach for a couple of reasons. First of all, the determination of which facts require documentation is almost wholly dependent upon one's beliefs. When a person believes an assertion to be undeniably true, he sees no need to substantiate it. If, however, he doubts the veracity of a statement, he is likely to demand some kind of validation. What complicates matters is that beliefs—even those considered to be fundamental truths—differ markedly among individuals. If I had attempted to validate every statement that someone might question, the Notes section would be almost as long as the text! Here is the guideline I used for providing documentation: For information I acquired directly from a particular source, I included an endnote to credit that source. For knowledge I've gleaned from multiple sources over the years, I did not include an endnote.

The second reason for not providing supporting data for every statement that might be questioned is that including such corroboration wouldn't really prove anything. Physicists have discovered that simply observing an atom or subatomic particle changes its behavior.[1] Since everything in our reality is composed of atoms, *everything* is influenced by the observer! Experiments and studies (including double-blind studies) are affected by the beliefs, perceptions, and expectations of the people involved. Therefore, even "conclusively proven" scientific findings may not be (and often aren't) any more valid than what your grandmother told you when you were a child.

It's likely that some of the information in this book will challenge your beliefs—and it is meant to. Certain ideas may even seem preposterous to you. However, I encourage you not to let that stop you from making use of the information you do find helpful. Personally, I've learned not to dismiss or discount everything a person has to offer simply because I disagree with him or her in certain areas. (In fact, in most of the books I reference and/or recommend, I don't agree with *all* of the authors' ideas.) Each of us views the world through the filters of our own beliefs, and no one is infallible. Keep in mind that I'm simply offering information, not trying to convince anyone that my views are the "right" ones. Use whatever is helpful to you, and mentally set aside the rest.

My intention is to help you become aware that there is an alternative to the dismal path you've seen so many people (possibly your own parents) follow: progressive physical and mental degeneration leading to suffering, loss of function, and an unpleasant death. Until now, scientists (and most of us) have viewed the physical body as much like an automobile you were randomly assigned—the best you can do is keep it running as well as possible as it gradually falls apart with age. *Transcend the Aging Process* presents an alternative viewpoint: that by changing the way you perceive your body and realizing that you are in control of its condition, you can dramatically alter the way you experience aging.

"I plan on growing old much later in life, or maybe not at all."

—Patty Carey

PART I
Paradigm Shift

1

The New View of Aging

"*Problems cannot be solved at the same level of awareness that created them.*"

—*Albert Einstein*

Old Ideas About Aging

If you take a look at a newsstand, you may notice an interesting trend: magazine articles about anti-aging are starting to outnumber those on weight loss. Several best-selling books promise lifelong youth, or at least the appearance of it. Advertising for anti-aging products is becoming even more prevalent. Companies promote skin care products, hair growth formulas, nutritional supplements, pharmaceutical drugs, and even pantyhose as solutions to the problems of aging. Anti-aging is a multibillion dollar industry, and the trend isn't likely to slow down anytime soon. In the United States, one of the most youth-oriented cultures in the world, another person turns 50 every few seconds.

In my observation, people who have reached an age when they start worrying about getting older generally fall into four groups. The first group consists of those who are resigned to the "fact" that they will degenerate with age, and they're trying to manage their growing health problems with medical treatments. They enjoy discussing their various ailments and make frequent references to their declining mental and physical condition. To hear some of them talk, you'd think they were 100 years old, when in fact they are closer to half that age. In the more extreme cases, the person's life revolves around doctor visits, surgical operations, and prescription drugs. Their infirmities have become a significant part of their personality.

Members of the second group also believe it is natural to deteriorate with age, but they're determined to fight it with diet, exercise, nutritional and hormone supplements, skin care products, plastic surgery, and anything else they think might help. They stay informed about anti-aging research and are eagerly awaiting the next scientific breakthrough or product that will provide "the answer." Compared to the first group, most members of the second group are in very good health. Slim, fit, and active, they often appear younger than their contemporaries. However, most of them work hard at it and spend a great deal of money on dietary supplements, cosmetic treatments, and health club memberships. Some of them take so many pills every day that it's surprising they don't rattle when they do their aerobic exercise. (If it seems I'm being unduly harsh on this group, it's because I spent so many years as a member of it!)

The third group combines the characteristics of the first two groups but is considerably less extreme than either of them. Members of this group expect to gradually deteriorate with age, but they don't focus on it a great deal. They make an effort to take care of their health in conventional ways such as having regular medical checkups, getting some exercise, taking a multivitamin supplement, and so forth. Beyond these basic measures, they don't believe there is much they can do to prevent the eventual breakdown of their body. Many of them are dealing with aging parents who require special care. The idea that they might end up in the same position as their parents makes them uneasy, so they try to avoid thinking about it.

The fourth group (at this point, it's by far the smallest of the groups) understands that age-related degeneration is not inevitable; it is the result of aligning with a belief system. They don't accept the conventional idea that their future is dictated by genetics or external factors. Most members of this group use medical services or pharmaceutical drugs infrequently (if at all) and don't spend much money on nutritional supplements or cosmetic treatments. This is not to say that many of them don't exercise, eat nutritious foods, and take care of their body. It's simply that they realize these external activities are not what keeps them healthy and youthful.

What is most impressive about the people in the fourth group is that—regardless of their genetics—they aren't aging at the same rate as their contemporaries. "My genetic heritage suggests I would have female reproductive problems such as breast cancer and fibroid [uterine] tumors, probably resulting in a hysterectomy by age 45," said Marcy, now in her early fifties. "My family history also indicates I'd have heart disease, chronic depression, and sinus trouble, and that I would be overweight in middle age. I have none of these health problems, and I'm not overweight," she noted. She has no dental problems and hasn't been to a dentist since age 14. "The last time I had a gynecological exam, the nurse said I was the oldest patient they'd seen all day—and also the healthiest," remarked Marcy, who looks considerably younger than most people her age. And although she has been nearsighted since childhood, she doesn't need bifocals. "I went to the eye doctor the other day, and he said I have very 'youthful' eyes. Even my astigmatism has cleared up," Marcy added.

It isn't uncommon for those in the fourth group to be taken for 10 or 15 years younger than their chronological age. A couple of years ago, I was discussing Chinese astrology with a young-looking man who mentioned that he was born in the Year of the Snake. I assumed he meant 1965, and was shocked to discover that his birth date actually was 12 years earlier (Chinese zodiac signs recur every 12 years). When I met my friend John, he mentioned that he was born in 1953, but he looked so much younger that I assumed he meant 1963. I was so sure I'd misheard him that I asked him to repeat himself three times! John has excellent health and almost never gets sick (even with minor illnesses), does not wear glasses, and hasn't been to a doctor in several years. He takes no drugs or nutritional supplements other than a vegetable-based green drink every other day and an occasional vitamin C tablet. John exercises only moderately (some calisthenics and about 30 minutes of aerobic exercise three times a week), yet he can walk and climb at high altitudes with greater endurance than most people, even those much younger.

While writing this book, I met a beautiful, youthful, and vibrant woman of indeterminate age. Since she obviously took good care of herself, I guessed Barbara to be in her early fifties, although she gave the impression of someone younger. Later I learned she was in her mid-sixties, in excellent health, and hadn't had any cosmetic surgery. I'm not the only one who assumed Barbara was much younger than her chronological age. A male friend of hers, eight years her junior, said one of his clients saw a picture of the two of them together and asked if Barbara was his daughter! At a grocery store recently, Barbara requested the senior citizens' discount (for customers age 60 and older) and the clerk laughed, assuming she was joking. In a reverse version of being "carded," Barbara was asked to produce her driver's license to prove she was entitled to the discount. The astonished clerk exclaimed, "You look *great*! I sure hope I look that good when I'm older."

At this point, you may be wondering what is the secret of people in the fourth group—have they discovered the fountain of youth? In a way, perhaps they have. Those in the fourth group do not align with the conventional belief that age-related degeneration is inevitable. Rather, they realize that how they experience growing older is primarily determined by their own beliefs and choices.

The burgeoning anti-aging industry has been operating from a flawed premise: that degeneration is a natural part of aging built into our DNA. The truth is that cell behavior is controlled not by our genes, but by our perceptions of (and reactions to) the environment. In other words, *we* control the aging process.

A New Paradigm

According to conventional beliefs about aging, we're on a countdown clock to degeneration and the best we can do is try to hold things together as long as possible. Conventional medical science views the human body as fundamentally defective—if left to its own devices, it will deteriorate with age until it can no longer function. Anti-aging researchers study the mechanics of the aging process: DNA transcription errors, cells that no longer replicate after a finite number of divisions, organ function that deteriorates over time, and so forth. The goal is to find out what goes wrong that causes age-related degeneration and to develop methods of outsmarting the body to prevent these changes from occurring.

Within a narrow context, this view seems to be correct, but it's only part of the story—a very limited part. The scientific perception of the human body as a flawed piece of machinery that breaks down over time flies in the face of the spiritual view of humans as perfectly created beings. A person is not just a physical body and brain with consciousness tacked on as an afterthought. The mechanistic view of the human body is inaccurate—consciousness creates the physical body, not the other way around. The physical form is simply a manifestation of a nonphysical being.

It isn't necessarily that anti-aging researchers are barking up the wrong tree; many of the trees they're looking in actually do have something there. The problem is that they're focusing on the trees without even noticing the forest. Many of the current theories point to free radicals as a primary cause of age-related degeneration. (Free radicals are oxygen molecules that have lost an electron and stabilize themselves by taking an electron from a nearby molecule, which causes cell damage.) What the researchers fail to recognize is that we don't age because our bodies produce too many free radicals—we produce too many free radicals because we believe in aging.

The fundamental reason for age-related degeneration is not that the body is defective; it is that we essentially *program* it to decline with age. What if we expected to continue functioning at an optimal level, provided the nutrients, water, rest, and exercise to enable our cells to do their jobs properly, and did our best to avoid exposure to toxins? It's very likely we would discover that most of the detrimental age-related changes would not occur. Change is inevitable, but deterioration is not. It is possible to function optimally into old age—without high-technology medical intervention.

This is not to say we would continue to look exactly as we did at age 25 if we simply altered our beliefs about aging. The body is a reflection of our inner self, which changes in every moment. I doubt that many people would want to stay exactly as they were in their youth, with the same attitudes and maturity level they possessed at 25. As we become more experienced and acquire wisdom, it's natural to project a physical image that appears older. Some people may say, "I'd love to be able to keep the wisdom, knowledge, and skills I've attained, yet look like I did when I was 20." But would they really? I suspect that most adults with a fair number of years of experience want to be recognized as a little older because it draws more credibility and respect, at least in our society. A 50-year-old lawyer, for instance, probably wants to be acknowledged as more experienced than her 25-year-old colleague. Youth certainly has its charm, but the more defined features of a full-fledged adult can be more attractive than the somewhat unformed features of an 18-year-old.

Change is natural, but that doesn't mean we have to start falling apart when we reach a particular age. The primary reason people deteriorate with age is that they believe they will. Our physical form is a manifestation of our nonphysical self, and it does what we expect it to do. If an authority figure like a scientist or doctor tells people they will degenerate because they have reached a certain age, then they are likely to believe it—and will do just that. Our beliefs and perceptions cause electrical and chemical reactions in our bodies. If you believe your body is breaking down, you will *cause* it to break down. It's much like when a physician tells a patient he has three months left to live and the patient dies precisely three months later, or when a witch doctor puts a curse on a person and it works. (The "witch doctors" in our culture usually have medical degrees.)

Your body is not a vehicle you inhabit; it is a creation of your nonphysical being and therefore reflects your personality characteristics. Facial wrinkles (expression lines) may be an external manifestation of people's automatic reactions—habitually doing the same things and repeatedly making the same choices. An inflexible body can be a physical representation of becoming set in one's ways. Many people become less mentally flexible as they get older, hence the stiffness and loss of physical flexibility experienced by so many older adults. It can happen the other way around as well: if we become more mentally flexible, our physical flexibility can increase. I'm living proof that this is possible. When I was younger, I was quite rigid in my attitudes and physically inflexible as well. Not surprisingly, I disliked stretching exercises. Contrary to what is expected to occur as we age, my physical flexibility has increased considerably, and I now enjoy stretching exercises.

Many people consider the words *mind* and *brain* to be almost synonymous, and they believe the mind resides in the brain. It doesn't. The mind exists in the energy field that surrounds, permeates, and in fact *creates* our physical body and brain. In addition, the mind—and therefore the personality—does not die when the body ceases to function.

The mind-body effect is not hocus-pocus; it's an actual physiological process. If you doubt that your perceptions and beliefs can affect your body, just think of what happens when you hear something upsetting. If, for example, someone told you one of your loved ones was in a serious accident, you would experience immediate physiological changes. Your heart would start beating faster (raising your blood pressure and pulse rate), your breathing would quicken, and you might break out in a sweat. Nothing really happened to you, so what caused all these changes? Simply your perceptions, beliefs, and thoughts! Most of us don't realize that what we think and speak affects our body. Each time you think or say something like, "I forgot where I put my car keys again. I must be getting old," you are reinforcing a belief that tells your body you expect it to deteriorate. Such reinforcement has a cumulative effect, which is why the people who think and talk the most about getting old are the ones who seem to age the fastest.

Behind these thoughts of aging and degeneration are *beliefs*. Most of us have grown up in an environment where we not only see people deteriorating with age, we are taught that it's a normal part of life that cannot be avoided. Therefore our brains and bodies, like obedient little soldiers, react to our beliefs and give us exactly what we're asking for. Fortunately, it doesn't have to be this way. Once we realize that our perceptions and beliefs are the primary cause of physical and mental degeneration, we can make a choice to align with different beliefs.

Think of your body as if it were a corporation: your mind is the chief executive officer (CEO), the organ systems are the divisions, the organs are the departments, and the cells are the workers. The workers, departments, and divisions all try to do a good job and satisfy the CEO. The CEO, however, often is unclear about what he wants and gives mixed messages to his employees. He expects them to do one thing (in this case, deteriorate with age), and then complains about it when they meet his expectations. Also, he often does not supply the workers with the proper materials (nutrients and water) to run the factory, adequate rest breaks (sleep), and activity periods (exercise), yet he expects them to continue performing at an optimal level and becomes angry when they don't. The CEO then calls in experts (health care professionals) to find ways to deal with the "problematic" employees. In truth, the workers are not the problem; they are merely doing what the CEO indicates he wants them to do.

The Biology of Belief

All of this sounds great, you may be thinking, but why isn't there scientific evidence to substantiate it? Ah, but there *is* scientific evidence. Cellular biologist Bruce H. Lipton, Ph.D. has shown that the health and behavior of our cells is controlled not by our genes, but by our environment—or more specifically, by our *reactions* to the environment. Although Dr. Lipton's research is not directed towards the study of human aging, I recognized that his research is pertinent to that subject. It should be noted, however, that the conclusions drawn in this book about the relationship of Dr. Lipton's findings to human aging are my own.

Bruce Lipton's work first came to my attention when I attended his presentation at a conference in September 1999. As it ended, I sat dumbfounded and declared to a friend, "This presentation has changed my life." Melodramatic, but true. From years of studying metaphysics, I had learned that we create our own reality, but there was a part of me—the logical, rational part—that needed to understand *how*. Finally, in terms I could comprehend, was an explanation that filled the gap. And it came from a highly credible source: a cellular biologist with impressive credentials. Bruce Lipton received his doctorate from the University of Virginia, has served on the faculty of several medical schools, and spent five years as a research fellow at Stanford University's School of Medicine.

Dr. Lipton's research revealed that scientists have been making logical conclusions based on a fundamentally flawed premise: that the characteristics and fate of a life form are dependent upon its genes. If the brain is removed from an organism, the organism immediately dies. Removing a cell's nucleus (which contains the DNA and hence the genes) does not kill the cell, which proves that the nucleus is not the cell's command center or "brain," as is commonly believed. According to Dr. Lipton, "If the nucleus truly represented the brain of the cell, then removal of the nucleus would result in the cessation of cell functions and immediate cell death. However, experimentally enucleated [with the nucleus removed] cells may survive for two or more months without genes, and yet are capable of effecting complex responses to environmental and cytoplasmic stimuli.

Logic reveals that the nucleus *cannot* be the brain of the cell!"[2] This finding proves that genetic determinism (the idea that the characteristics of an organism are determined by its genes) is a myth.

Through studies on cloned human cells, Lipton recognized that the cell's "brain" is actually the cell membrane. The cell membrane, which separates the cell from the external environment, was the first biological organelle (structure within a cell that performs a differentiated function) to appear in evolution, and it is the only organelle common to every living organism.

Cell membranes are composed primarily of phospholipids (major structural lipids, or fats) and proteins, including special proteins called Integral Membrane Proteins (IMPs). The two types of IMPs are receptors, the "sense organs" of the cell, and effectors, which carry out cell behavior. According to Lipton, "Receptor IMPs 'see' or are 'aware' of their environment, and effector IMPs create physical responses that translate environmental signals into an appropriate biological behavior. The IMP complex *controls* behavior, and through its effect upon regulatory proteins, these IMPs also control gene expression… The IMP complexes provide the cell with 'awareness of the environment through physical sensation,' which by dictionary definition represents *perception*. Each receptor-effector protein complex collectively constitutes a 'unit of perception.'"[3]

Scientists traditionally believed receptors responded only to molecules (matter), but new research has shown that receptors also respond to energy signals. "Conventional medicine has consistently ignored research published in its own mainstream scientific journals, research that clearly reveals the regulatory influence that electromagnetic fields have on cell physiology," notes Lipton. "Pulsed electromagnetic fields have been shown to regulate virtually every cell function, including DNA synthesis, RNA synthesis, protein synthesis, cell division, cell differentiation, morphogenesis, and neuroendocrine regulation. These findings are relevant, for they acknowledge that biological behavior can be controlled by 'invisible' energy forces, which include *thought*."[4]

One of Bruce Lipton's fundamental concepts is that a cell can be in only one of two modes: growth or protection. *Growth* in this context can also be described as love, openness, and expansion; *protection* equates to fear, closure, and contraction. When we perceive our environment to be dangerous, our cells go into protection mode and fail to use available resources to rebuild, repair, and renew.

Growth and protection also can be associated with anabolism (rebuild and repair processes) and catabolism (breakdown processes) According to the metabolic theory of aging,[5] degeneration occurs when the body's catabolic processes exceed the anabolic processes. We all start out as highly anabolic, but conventional science says the ratio naturally changes as we grow older—catabolic processes become increasingly dominant, resulting in the degeneration we call aging.

From Dr. Lipton's research, I learned that whether we are in growth or protection mode depends upon our perceptions of (and reactions to) the environment. Applied to the metabolic theory of aging, this means that developing an increasingly catabolic metabolism as we grow older is not inevitable. Anabolism equals growth. If we perceive our environment to be safe, our cells will be in growth rather than protection mode, resulting in a metabolism that is more anabolic than catabolic. *Therefore, we—not our genes—control the rate at which our bodies age.*

Bruce Lipton's research (and his tireless efforts to share this information with others) is playing an important role in advancing our understanding of the nature of reality. For more information about Dr. Lipton's work, refer to his website (*www.brucelipton.com*) or contact Spirit 2000, Inc. by mail at P.O. Box 41126, Memphis, Tennessee 38174 USA; by phone at 1-800-245-9463 (toll-free); or online at *www.spirit2000.com*.

Your Body Reflects Your Beliefs

Inflammation (an immune system response) is implicated in numerous age-associated disorders such as arthritis, diabetes, cancer, heart disease, and Alzheimer's disease. It has long been known to play a role in allergies and asthma, as well as autoimmune diseases such as lupus and multiple sclerosis, in which the immune system attacks the body's own tissues as if they were foreign invaders.

The immune system is the body's defense system, and like all defense systems, it is activated when a threat is perceived. Whether the threat is real or not is immaterial; it is the *perception* of danger that triggers the immune response. Therefore, it is conceivable that the fundamental precipitating factor in many diverse age-associated disorders is *fear*. In our society, it's typical for people to live in a state of low-grade, constant fear. Most news reports and much of our advertising is fear-based. Years of exposure to these fear-inducing stimuli may activate the immune system and cause inflammation, which eventually damages the tissues enough to result in an obvious disease state.

The physical effects of beliefs and expectations were clearly demonstrated in an experiment performed by psychologist Shlomo Breznitz at Hebrew University, Jerusalem.[6] Breznitz had several groups of Israeli soldiers march 40 kilometers (about 25 miles), but gave conflicting information to each group. Some groups marched 30 kilometers and then were told they had to march 10 more. Others were told they would march 60 kilometers, but actually marched only 40. Some groups were allowed to see distance markers; others had no external means of gauging the distance they had walked. After the soldiers completed the marches, Breznitz measured their blood levels of stress hormones and found significant differences among the groups, even though they all had walked the same distance. The soldiers' hormone levels clearly reflected their *beliefs and perceptions* about the distances they marched rather the actual distances. The findings of this experiment (and many others like it) have significant implications regarding how we experience the aging process. Our beliefs about what to expect as we get older not only have tangible, measurable effects on our physiology, they actually define our experience of aging.

Personally, my experience of physical aging has followed my expectations almost precisely. I haven't experienced most of the age-related changes many of my contemporaries report because I did not expect to, and the changes I've noticed are those I believed would occur. A good example is gray hair. My mother and her sisters started getting gray hair in their early twenties; my father's hair began to turn gray in his forties. I didn't think I would get gray hair quite as early as my mother, but figured that due to heredity, I'd surely have it in my thirties. Not surprisingly, by my mid-thirties I had a noticeable quantity of silver strands. Not only did I expect gray hair, I sometimes remarked that I was surprised I didn't get it even earlier, since it runs in my family. Ironically, at a recent family reunion, I noted that my three older siblings all have significantly less gray hair than I do. In fact, each of them has less gray hair than most people their age—hardly enough to even notice. The four of us have the same parents and therefore share the heredity in which gray hair "runs in the family." The difference is that I expected to develop gray hair at an early age and they did not. My gray hair was due not to heredity, but to my belief in the influence of heredity.

In his book *Past Fear and Doubt to Amazing Abundance*, Stephen Hawley Martin shares a thought-provoking experience he had in a 7-Eleven convenience store.[7] While waiting in line to buy a bottle of beer, he noticed a sign that said, "We I.D. Under 27 Years of Age." When Martin reached the counter, the clerk requested his identification. At first he thought she was joking, but the clerk told him she was quite serious, so he produced his driver's license. The woman gasped in amazement when she saw his birth date, which revealed that he was 55 years old—more than twice the age required to show identification to purchase alcohol.

Not only did the clerk think he looked no older than 27, Martin realized he felt just as young as he had at that age. Pondering the incident later, he recalled that when he was 25, he read an article about a study that found that people who took large doses of vitamin E did not show any measurable signs of aging. Thinking that vitamin E was a veritable fountain of youth, he bought a bottle and had continued taking it ever since, truly believing the pills would keep him from aging. Quite a few years later, he saw another article that said vitamin E supplements could not be proven to retard aging, but he dismissed the study results and continued taking it anyway. Although subsequent research has shown that vitamin E supplementation does appear to lower the incidence of cardiovascular disease, cancer, and other health problems, it clearly has not prevented its users from showing any signs of aging. After the incident in the convenience store, Martin realized that very likely, the vitamin E supplement had worked for him largely due to the placebo effect.

Martin's experience with vitamin E supplements is similar to what happened to me when I took gelatin for my fingernails. At age 10, I had weak fingernails that cracked and peeled easily. I wanted my nails to be strong so I could grow them long like my aunt, who had beautiful nails. When I asked her for advice, she told me she drank gelatin daily to strengthen her nails. I started drinking the nasty stuff every day as well, and within a few months my nails became quite strong and were growing faster. I continued taking gelatin for about three years, but even after I quit taking it, my nails stayed strong and grew quickly. By that time, I had come to think of myself as a person with naturally strong nails. I now prefer to keep my nails short, but when I want to grow them long, I can do so easily. Many years after my gelatin-drinking days, I learned that consuming gelatin has no effect whatsoever on fingernails—the substance is just incomplete, inferior protein. It was my belief in the product that made my nails strong, not the product itself.

Stories about the placebo effect abound. Psychotherapist Robert M. Williams, M.A. relates a particularly poignant one in his book, *The Missing (Piece) Peace in Your Life.*[8] In the late 1980s, an Eastern European family that had emigrated to the United States sent a large "care package" to their relatives back home who were having difficulty obtaining basic supplies. Communications were slow, so it was nearly six months before the family received a letter from the appreciative recipients. The relatives said they were most grateful for the medication, which had helped numerous family members experience significant improvements in their health. The medication was running low, and they were fervently requesting more. Those who assembled the care package were puzzled—no one remembered having sent any medication. Ultimately they discovered that the "medication" was actually a popular candy! "Please, please send more of the Lifesavers," their relatives entreated. "They made such a difference!"

Why Does Aging Occur?

I have identified four basic reasons we experience the changes we call aging:

1. Belief in the negative aspects of growing older and the expectation that the body and brain will deteriorate over time.

2. Habitually existing in protection mode rather than growth mode: fear, contraction, and choking off one's life energy.

3. Belief in the effects of health-related factors such as lack of adequate nutrients and exercise, as well as exposure to substances and conditions believed to have detrimental effects on the human body. These factors influence us only because of our belief that they do, but these beliefs are widely held and deeply entrenched.

4. Changes to our inner self that are reflected in our physical countenance: we feel older; therefore we look older. However, these changes can manifest as subtle alterations rather than the obvious signs of degeneration we've learned to expect.

The good news is that we can directly influence the first three factors, reducing undesirable aging-related changes to a minimum.

2

Limiting Beliefs About Aging

○ ○
"Ah, but I was so much older then; I'm younger than that now."
—*Bob Dylan*[9]

Consciousness Shift

There is a shift in human consciousness occurring now, a movement to a state of greater awareness. Part of this shift is recognizing that what we consider to be absolutes—the concepts we've based our world upon—are simply beliefs we choose to align with, not unalterable truths. In other words, we made the rules and then forgot we did, and now slavishly follow these rules as if we had no other choice. How tenaciously we cling to our narrow definitions of what we believe constitutes reality!

Many people sense this shift in consciousness but don't really understand it. Rather than recognizing that virtually all of our fundamental institutions—including science and religion—are based upon belief systems, some of us are creating additional beliefs to explain the consciousness shift. Those who abandon traditional religions for New Age alternatives are typically just swapping one set of beliefs for another. They still are looking for something outside of themselves to provide "the answer," but now it's astrology instead of psychology, a guru in lieu of a priest.

Beliefs and Truths

In our reality, there are no absolute truths. (That statement itself is an absolute, but it's the best I can do within the limitations of our language.) Virtually everything we consider to be a truth is actually a belief. We take on most of our cultural and familial beliefs in early childhood—automatically, as if by osmosis. Usually we aren't even aware that they are beliefs; we think of them as principles that define "the way things really are." These fundamental beliefs become our personal truths—the basis on which we determine whether something is good or bad, true or false, or right or wrong. Contrary to what most of us have been taught, beliefs are not a matter of right or wrong; they're simply preferences.

The key to transformational personal growth is realizing that our "truths" are actually beliefs, which means they are subject to change—and to choice. If you aren't happy with something (in this case, age-related degeneration or the anticipation of it), you can choose to align with a different belief, and this will change your experience. Many age-related beliefs are commonly accepted as truths. How often have you heard (or made) statements like, "He looks good for his age," or expressed surprise that a 60-year-old woman ran a marathon? We may want to believe that getting older means getting better, but our thoughts and words reveal our true beliefs.

In an example of how differently we tend to perceive ourselves at different ages, recently a 12-year-old friend was having difficulty accessing an Internet account. At first she assumed the problem was that she'd forgotten her password, but after three days of struggling with the account, she realized she had been misspelling her user name. The girl berated herself for being stupid, which I assured her was not the case. Her user name was 14 letters long and had a strange spelling; it would be easy for anyone to get it wrong.

If my friend had been 42 or 52 instead of 12, it's likely she would have attributed the error not to a lack of intelligence, but to encroaching senility or Alzheimer's disease. Think about how commonly we hear people say things like, "I forgot where I parked my car; I must be getting senile." Individuals of all ages do absent-minded things, not because they are stupid or their brain is deteriorating, but because they aren't paying attention (a subject that merits a book of its own). When I can't find my car in a parking lot, it isn't because I forgot where I parked it. The problem is that I never noticed in the first place.

You Control Your Body

We have the innate capability to maintain our physical bodies in a healthy and attractive state without any outside help (drugs, hormones, nutritional supplements, cosmetic procedures, and so forth). However, it can be difficult to alter an ingrained belief without some physical evidence that it's possible. When people make lifestyle adjustments that result in desirable physical changes such as increased energy, greater flexibility, better skin tone, and loss of excess fat, this helps to shift their beliefs about what is possible. But regardless of any drugs, supplements, exercises, cosmetic treatments, or anything else you may try, if you believe aging means deterioration, then ultimately you will deteriorate.

In altering my beliefs about aging, I've found it helpful to hear about people who have made physical changes not considered possible according our cultural belief systems. If you have difficulty accepting the idea that we can influence our physical bodies in profound ways, consider the implications of the following Dissociative Identity Disorder (DID) (formerly known as Multiple Personality Disorder) cases discussed in *The Holographic Universe*.[10]

A person diagnosed with DID has distinct subpersonalities, at least some of which are not aware of all the others. Not only are the personalities different, there can be dramatic biological differences between them. Allergies, for instance, often are present only in some of the personalities. In one DID case, all but one of a man's subpersonalities were allergic to orange juice and would develop a severe rash if they drank it. If the man switched to the nonallergic personality, the rash would immediately start receding, and he could drink orange juice with no problem.

Not only allergies, but also the effects of alcohol and medication can vary greatly among subpersonalities. A DID patient who is drunk may instantly become sober by switching personalities. If an adult personality is given an adult dose of medication and a child personality subsequently takes over, it sometimes results in an overdose. A DID patient may have to carry several pairs of eyeglasses due to substantial differences in vision among various personalities. In some women, each of the female subpersonalities has her own menstrual cycle. Even more surprising, some subpersonalities have different eye colors and voice patterns. (According to speech pathologists, even expert actors cannot alter their voice patterns.) Other conditions that may change from one subpersonality to the next include scars, cysts, color blindness, diabetes, epilepsy, and left-and right-handedness.

The fact that physical characteristics and conditions such as eye color, left-handedness, and diabetes can change from moment to moment in a DID patient means that physical characteristics are subject to change, not "hardwired" into us as we've been led to believe. If a DID patient can eliminate an allergy or metabolic disorder, then why can't anyone? When you realize that humans have the ability to change their eye color, then it isn't so hard to believe you can alter or avoid things like facial wrinkles, fat deposits, and failing vision.

Also, don't get caught in the trap of believing you are likely to inherit whatever disorders "run in your family." Genetic heritage may give you tendencies for certain traits, but you choose whether or not to actualize them. As Marcy (mentioned in Chapter 1) remarked, "I decided a long time ago that I was not like everyone else in my family, and that their physical problems had nothing to do with me—and they haven't. Even though my genetics probably has all the markers for those disorders, I decided not to align with the belief that I would inherit the family ills, so they were never activated." It is noteworthy that Marcy no longer goes for routine medical checkups and diagnostic tests. As she put it, "I decided that if I kept going for the exams, eventually they would 'find something.'"

Models of Youthfulness

In the Far East, there are numerous accounts of people who have maintained or regained youthful appearance and functioning well into old age. Nevertheless, I wanted to find at least a few individuals in Western cultures that have transcended negative beliefs about aging—people who could serve as examples to prove it can be done. The individuals would have to be old enough chronologically to obviously have not followed the norm (preferably, at least age 60). I haven't yet reached an age where I can serve as such an example.

The day I told a friend I wanted to find individuals who could demonstrate these concepts, I happened upon an advertisement for a book called *How Long Do You Choose to Live?* by Peter Ragnar.[11] The author, who describes himself as a "senior citizen, author, athlete, mentalist, and public speaker," apparently is living proof that my ideas about aging are valid. He is in perfect health, demonstrates impressive feats of strength and mental performance, and looks at least as young in a recent picture as he does in a photograph taken 18 years earlier. He has written several books, and other people have written books about him. I haven't met Peter Ragnar in person, but after reading his book and hearing recorded testimonials from many people who know him, I believe he has indeed broken out of the mold of limiting beliefs regarding aging. In the next few years, I expect to see an increasing number of individuals who have done the same thing.

Barbara, the woman mentioned in Chapter 1 who had to show her driver's license to get a senior citizen's discount, is another example of the new paradigm of aging. Barbara isn't in denial about her age; she loves being a grandmother, but also likes to dress stylishly and engage in active pursuits like dancing and skiing.

In every way but chronologically, she is younger than many people who are 20 years her junior. A key difference between Barbara and most of her contemporaries is that she *doesn't think of herself as old.*

Numerous well-known individuals are remaining youthful well beyond age 40, which used to be considered "over the hill." Media personality and producer Dick Clark has been recognized for his youthfulness as much as for his 50-year career of achievements in the television industry. Actress Sophia Loren, who has been starring in movies since the 1950s, is still stunningly beautiful. Fitness expert Jack La Lanne (born in 1914) is legendary for the feats of strength and endurance he continues to perform. A younger example is actress Rene Russo (born in the middle of the baby boom), whose perennial youthful beauty is reportedly not due to plastic surgery. In addition, some of the well-known personalities who have availed themselves of cosmetic procedures are staying more youthful overall than these procedures could account for on their own.

Long-term practitioners of yoga (an ancient Indian art based on a harmonizing system of development for the mind, body, and spirit) also typically remain more youthful than their contemporaries. Several years ago I read about a yoga instructor, an African-American woman who appeared to be in her late thirties, who was speaking to middle school students about the practice of yoga. Many of the students seemed unreceptive to her ideas; some were almost belligerent. When she asked them to guess her age, they intended to insult her by guessing she was in her fifties. When she revealed that she was over 70 years old and had been practicing and teaching yoga for more than 30 years, the students gave her their rapt attention for the rest of the presentation.

Celebrating Birthdays

The term *aging* itself is almost synonymous with degeneration. Whether applied to a human being or an inanimate object, it implies loss—loss of function, usefulness, attractiveness, and desirability. It would be helpful to use another word (at least in your own mind) to describe getting older. *Evolvement* is a good alternative, since it implies advancement in a positive way. You're not aging; you're evolving.

Our culture categorizes people by age so much that it's hard not to get sucked into conventional thinking, particularly when you have a "landmark" birthday with a number ending in zero. I've found it helpful to decide on alternate meanings for these occasions before they occur. Turning 50, for example, doesn't have to mean you are over the hill. It can mean you no longer have to follow rules or conventions that aren't to your liking (provided you're willing to face the consequences). At this point in your life, you may feel you've learned enough to know what is right for you and to make your own decisions. You probably will opt to continue to pay income taxes and such (there's that consequences thing), but you don't have to act like a person your age is "supposed" to act. You can dress like a teenager, ride a roller coaster and shriek like a banshee, stay up all night yakking with your best friend, or whatever else strikes your fancy. If you don't limit yourself to the expected behaviors for people born when you were, then you'll be less likely to fall into the conventional pattern and start manifesting the signs of physical and mental degeneration that also are expected to occur when you reach certain ages.

Shortly after a landmark birthday, I had an employer-required medical checkup and was amazed at the number of negative suggestions I received from health care professionals. They recommended numerous diagnostic tests, insinuating that—based only upon my birth date and gender—I was vulnerable to all sorts of dire diseases. With each refusal of an unpleasant-sounding test (can you believe I turned down an offer for a free colonoscopy?), I said to myself, "This doesn't apply to me. I'm not going to manifest these things." I chose to react to their warnings in much the same way as if they had been giving me a lecture about not stealing from the company: I listened politely, but knew it wasn't relevant to me. I'd no sooner get cancer than I would embezzle company funds. It's simply not something I'm going to do in this lifetime. Disease and deterioration doesn't just *happen* to us; it's a choice of experience that's based on our beliefs.

This is an appropriate place to mention that when I use the word *choice* regarding illness, injury, and other hardships, I don't mean that a person chooses these problems the way he might choose an ice cream cone: "Yes, I'd like some of that lung cancer, thank you very much. And while we're at it, can you throw in a little arthritis, some diabetes, and maybe a car accident on top?" The individual most likely didn't *want* to develop a disease or have an accident, but it was the inner choices he made—the things he chose to believe and focus upon—that manifested physically in these ways.

A remark sometimes made to a person having a birthday is, "You may think you're old, but you should be happy—right now you're the youngest you will ever be." This assertion isn't really true. For example, a person born on January 1, 1950 had his fiftieth birthday on January 1, 2000. On that date, his 20-year-old self (who was "born" in 1970) turned 30 years old. His 50-year-old self, however, was just "born" that day. Therefore, his 20-year-old self is actually older than his

50-year-old self! The self we create *in each moment* is younger than all of our supposedly younger selves. There is some distortion in this idea; in truth, everything is created in the present moment—including our 50-year-old self, 20-year-old self, and newborn self. Viewed in the context of our beliefs about chronological time, however, this idea can be useful for reframing our limiting ideas about aging.

Realigning "Old" Beliefs

Following are some suggestions that may help you realign your beliefs about aging and reinforce the belief that aging (degeneration) is a choice, not an inevitability:

- Pay attention to everything you think and say regarding aging, and identify the underlying beliefs you are expressing. For instance, you may notice that an acquaintance you haven't seen for a couple of years looks older than she did the last time you saw her. Does this make you wonder if you are looking older as well, or anticipate a future when you will deteriorate? Challenge the truth of these old beliefs with your new knowledge.

- Offer yourself alternatives to negative age-related thoughts and statements. For example, if you notice that an elderly relative is becoming increasingly frail, remind yourself that his physical expression is a reflection of his beliefs, not yours. If your relative has aligned with the "aging equals degeneration" mind-set so prevalent in our culture, it doesn't mean you must do the same. Remember that you are in control of the aging process and can choose not to experience physical and mental decline.

- Start thinking of your body as self-renewing—as regenerating rather than deteriorating. Don't monitor your face and body for age-related changes. The more attention you give to such features, the more of them are likely to appear. Instead, focus on the aspects of your appearance that make you feel good. On some days you'll perceive that you look and feel young; on other days it may be the opposite. Your physical body is a manifestation of your inner self, which is constantly changing. The way you look and feel today will not necessarily be the way you look and feel tomorrow (or five minutes from now) unless that is what you choose to create.

- Rather than categorizing yourself by your age group, start thinking of yourself as a generic adult—a grownup of indeterminate age. Quite simply, you are a physically mature human being rather than an infant, child, or adolescent—and you will remain in that category until you leave this life, regardless of how many years of experience you have. When you define yourself as a 38-year-old or a person over 50, it's hard not to be affected by conventional ideas of what a person that age is supposed to be like. For this reason, I prefer not to join age-based organizations.

- Drop the habit of mentioning your age or even thinking about it very often. When you mention your age to people, they perceive you through the filters of their beliefs about a person that age and reflect those beliefs back to you. If you prefer not to discuss your age, when someone asks how old you are, you can say something humorous like, "I don't know. I stopped counting after ___." Use any number that strikes your fancy. Numbers over 100 or under 20 usually have the greatest impact.

- Don't use age or infirmity as justification for your choices. People who use age or limiting physical conditions as an excuse to avoid doing things are headed down a slippery slope that ultimately can lead to degeneration—even incapacity. If you don't want to do something, be honest about it, both with yourself and with others. If you enjoyed an activity in the past but don't care for it now, give yourself permission to eliminate it from your life. If you force yourself to continue, you may well manifest an injury or illness that will give you a reason not to do it anymore. Using advancing age as justification is likely to cause or exacerbate signs of age-related degeneration.

- When celebrating other people's birthdays, refrain from making age-related jokes that reinforce pessimistic ideas about growing older. Avoid buying birthday cards with negative age-related messages, particularly those that refer to loss of attractiveness or mental function. These supposedly humorous greeting cards may seem inconsequential, but they reinforce the age-related beliefs that lead to degeneration.

In realigning my own beliefs about aging, I've found it helpful to avoid paying much attention to the mass media (television, newspapers, magazines, and so forth). The media (especially advertisements) reinforces beliefs about age-related degeneration and poor health, as well as fears about crime, terrorism, and disasters. Watching television is the most insidious because it puts people in a state of high receptivity—they are basically programmed to accept whatever input comes across the screen. Home entertainment centers with large-screen televisions and lifelike audio systems intensify this effect. Once you are aware of this form of programming, you can make a conscious choice not to participate in it.

PART II
Mind Matters

3

Developing Awareness

○ ○
"We don't see things as they are, we see them as we are."

—*Anaïs Nin*

Paying Attention

Our fast-paced society teaches us to focus our attention outward, as if what goes on inside is of little importance. In fact, it is just the opposite: we create internally and project our creations into the external, physical world. The internal and external creations happen simultaneously; it isn't "cause and effect" in the way we typically think of it. More accurately, it's a *correspondence*: our inner and outer (physical) worlds move in sync. When we don't pay attention to our inner world, we go through life like a blindfolded artist indiscriminately slopping paint on a canvas. When the artist looks at his creations, he's often disappointed (perhaps even horrified), yet it never occurs to him that he could remove the blindfold and pay attention to what he's painting while he is painting it.

Many of us feel our busy schedules and the demands of daily life leave no time for introspection, yet we feel chronically stressed and dissatisfied. It's easy to fall into the habit of living with mediocrity, assuming our lives will continue that way in the foreseeable future and not thinking about it too much. Essentially, we're on "automatic pilot" to a destination we haven't consciously chosen. This seems to happen most when we're very busy, paying attention to matters that are urgent but not really important. Some people live their entire lives this way, creating urgency so they won't have the time or energy to think about much else.

How do we change this unfulfilling way of living? The answer is simple but not easy. The key is to develop the habit of paying attention to what you are feeling, thinking, saying, and doing—and what your *motivation* is for your thoughts, words, and actions. A method I've found helpful is to frequently ask myself, "In this moment, does what I am engaged in (doing and/or thinking) help fulfill my intentions?" If not, I ask myself what I could be doing or thinking that would be more beneficial. Paying attention to the way you feel about something will help you determine if it is in harmony with your intentions. This method presupposes that you are aware of your intentions, which isn't always the case. Nevertheless, most of us can easily identify at least our short-term intentions.

Thought, Emotion, and Intuition

Our emotions, physical senses, and inner senses (including intuition and impulses) are avenues of communication—feedback on what we are creating. If you feel bad, it's a signal to alter what you are doing or thinking by making new choices. Pain (physical or emotional) is telling you that something needs to be changed.

The function of *thought* is to translate and interpret communications from the emotions and senses. Thought is often used inappropriately, to override rather than interpret communications. There are countless times when I've had a feeling or intuition that later turned out to be correct, but I "logic-ed" myself out of it and failed to take advantage of the insight. A good example is when a person is driving and has an impulse to take an alternate route. Rather than simply taking the other route, she tells herself it would be silly to do so because that road is longer and has more stoplights. She goes her usual way and encounters a traffic jam due to road construction or an accident. The habit of using logic to contradict inner communications is like a one-person version of the humorous question, "Are you going to believe what you see or what I tell you?" We tend to believe what we tell ourselves rather than what we perceive with our inner senses and physical senses.

It is widely recognized that in making decisions, our thoughts (rational mind) and emotions are sometimes in conflict. "Should I follow my head or follow my heart?" is a common dilemma. "Following the head" often means making a choice that seems logical but feels wrong. "Following the heart" entails choosing what we want at a particular time, which may not be the best choice. An example of following the head instead of the heart in a detrimental way is a woman from a wealthy family who is smitten with a working-class man, but to please her parents she marries a rich man she doesn't love. However, marrying the working-class man may not be the best course of action either. The optimal decision might be to hold off on marrying either of them. Unbeknownst to her at this point, in six months the woman will meet and fall in love with a man who has a background similar to hers. Had she married the working-class man, after the first blush of passion wore off, their markedly different lifestyle preferences would have caused serious problems between them.

In this example, the woman's inner feelings—her intuition—almost surely would be telling her to wait, but she might override these feelings with emotions or logic. In decision-making, there are three things at play: logic, emotions, and intuition. Logic takes into account any facts we are aware of, information provided by our physical senses, and knowledge from past experiences—all of which is filtered through our beliefs. Emotions also are strongly affected by beliefs (for example, if we believe something will hurt us, then we're likely to be afraid of it), as well as by desires and preferences. Although intuition is often described as a feeling, it's quite different from emotions. Intuition is a communication from our inner self that is meant to steer us in the right direction to fulfill our life intentions.

Intuition sometimes conflicts with logic, emotions, or both. Logic is a useful tool, but it operates from limited information: only the facts we are consciously aware of (or paying attention to) at the time. Intuition takes into account information we may not be aware of yet, as well as the broader view of our fundamental life intentions. Emotions typically reflect what we want at a particular time, which may not be the best choice for us. Intuition usually is subtle, a small voice deep within you. Emotions, which tend to be out front yelling loudly, can easily drown out intuition's quiet voice. (This is not to say that emotions aren't necessary or useful; emotions are a fundamental method of human expression and an important avenue of communication.)

There have been times in my life when I've done something I didn't really want to do and that didn't make sense rationally, yet I felt compelled to do it. Later I would discover why, and it would be obvious I'd done the right thing at the right time. For example, on several occasions I've felt compelled to go somewhere I didn't want to go, with no logical reason for doing so. I'd be driving down the road while saying to myself, "Why am I going here? I have no reason to go here, and I don't even *want* to go!" Almost invariably, it turned out that I would "happen" to find something I'd been looking for or meet someone I needed to talk with. I suspect I've avoided some car accidents that way as well.

It takes practice to become skilled at discerning intuition's subtle communications from emotion's blatant signals. Individuals perceive intuition in diverse ways. It can manifest as an inner feeling, a thought or mental "flash," a voice in one's mind, or a physical sensation. Some people experience all these forms of communication at different times. Over time, you will become familiar with your own "language" of inner communications. The challenge is to get in touch with your intuition and listen to it even when it conflicts with emotions, logic, or both. In my experience, that little voice has *never* been wrong.

Making Choices

When you need to make a decision and are having trouble distinguishing intuition from emotions and logic, it's helpful to use an efficient method for choosing the best option. The most consistently reliable method for me is the "pick the choice that looks brighter" technique. I imagine myself doing whatever I would be doing if I made choice A, then I try it with choice B, and so on. Usually one scenario will look brighter than the others, which lets me know it's the best option.

Another method I often use is to formulate a yes-or-no question that captures the essence of the dilemma. I then imagine the words *yes* and *no* in different colors, in block letters on a blank white background. Usually for me the *yes* is red and the *no* is blue, but you may prefer to use other colors (perhaps green and red, like traffic lights). Both words start out fairly small, but then one of them will keep getting larger until it dominates the picture, giving me the answer.

Meditation

Sometimes I feel as if my conscious mind is an unruly, barking dog that needs to be put in the backyard so I can hear what my inner self has to say. Meditation (focused awareness) is an effective way of enhancing this inner communication, as well as reducing stress and achieving deep relaxation. Following a regular practice of meditation can be challenging for those who grew up in Western cultures, however. The most well-known form of meditation—maintaining a thought-free state for an extended period of time—requires the ability to calm and focus the mind, which isn't easy for everyone. Rather than trying to stop your thoughts, concentrate on something—perhaps a word (mantra), an image, or your breath. The type of meditation known as *mindfulness* (paying attention to what you are doing in the moment, without having extraneous thoughts) may be easier for some people.

Rather than considering meditation to be one more thing you have to do every day, think of it as a way of giving yourself (and your mind) a rest. The more enjoyable you can make your meditation practice, the more likely you will be to continue it. If you aren't accustomed to meditating and tend to have trouble staying still, start out with short sessions and gradually work up to longer ones. If you can't manage a 15-minute meditation period, then try meditating twice a day for just five minutes each time. Forcing yourself to meditate for longer than you are comfortable will make you dread the next session, which is why I don't recommend meditation practices that involve sitting in an uncomfortable position or forcing yourself to keep your eyes open. Meditation should help achieve a state of focused awareness that is relaxing, not unpleasant.

Meditation's Effect on Adrenal Hormones

In addition to numerous benefits such as deep relaxation and enhanced concentration ability, a regular meditation practice reduces blood levels of cortisol, the major adrenal cortex hormone. An integral part of the "fight or flight" response, cortisol is secreted in greater quantities in response to stress. When levels of the hormone are elevated for sustained periods of time, it can be detrimental to the body and brain.

The adrenal glands also produce another hormone believed to play an important role in aging: dehydroepiandosterone (DHEA), a steroid that can be converted into other steroid hormones such as estrogen and testosterone. DHEA has been dubbed the "youth hormone" because it is believed to counteract some of the biological effects of age-related degeneration. This hormone is considered a biomarker for aging because levels generally drop in proportion to a person's age. DHEA levels are high in young people, but usually decline markedly as a person gets older. A 70-year-old, for instance, may be producing only one-tenth of the DHEA he or she produced at age 25. Low levels of DHEA are directly correlated to depression, Alzheimer's disease, heart disease, and a host of other age-associated disorders.

The adrenal glands secrete DHEA in inverse proportion to cortisol: the more cortisol, the less DHEA. Logically it would seem that reducing the production of cortisol would lead to increased level of DHEA, and apparently it does. Several studies have shown that people who practice meditation have significantly higher DHEA levels than nonmeditators of the same age. In one study, researchers found that people who practiced Transcendental Meditation for 20 minutes twice a day had DHEA levels typically found in nonmeditators 5 to 10 years younger.[12]

DHEA can be taken in supplement form, and many people have used it without apparent ill effects—at least so far. Although it is sold in some natural foods stores along with the vitamin and herbal supplements, DHEA is a hormone—a drug, not a nutrient. With virtually all hormones, taking a supplement eventually results in the body lowering its own production of that hormone. I find it difficult to believe this won't happen with DHEA as well. There are no truly long-term studies of the effects of DHEA supplementation because no one has been taking it for more than a few years. Those who choose to try DHEA supplements should get a blood test to determine their current level of DHEA before deciding on a dosage. Also, taking the hormone intermittently rather than continuously reduces the likelihood that the body will become habituated to it.

Breathing

Far more attention is given to health concerns such as diet and exercise than to the seemingly simple activity of breathing. Considering that humans can survive for weeks without food and days without water, this attention seems a bit misplaced. Without air, we would perish in minutes. Yet many people are shallow breathers who rarely take full, deep breaths. One of the reasons physical exercise is so beneficial is that it forces us to breathe deeply.

It's worthwhile to spend a few minutes every day focusing on the breath. A good time to do this is after exercising or just before meditation. Following is a simple breathing technique that most people (those without serious respiratory problems) find easy and refreshing.

1. Sit or stand comfortably with your back straight. Throughout the exercise, keep your mouth closed.
2. To a slow count of four (about four seconds), take in a full, deep breath through your nose. Don't strain or try to pack in as much air as possible; just inhale until your lungs feel comfortably full. As you inhale, your chest and abdomen should expand.
3. Hold the breath for four seconds.
4. Exhale through your nose to a slow count of six (about six seconds).
5. Hold for two seconds.
6. Repeat the four-step cycle 10 times.

7. As you get used to doing this exercise, you can gradually increase the length of time between breaths (steps 2 and 4), but never to the point that you're straining yourself.

In the book *Breathing: Expanding Your Power and Energy*, author Michael Sky gives instructions for simple breathing exercises and explains how breathing relates to emotional responses, interpersonal communication, and the movement of life force energy in the body.[13] According to Sky, constricting the breath is an instinctive response to physical or emotional discomfort. Most of us develop the habit of constricting our breath very early in life (typically from birth), which restricts the movement of energy in the body and keeps us mired in old patterns. A technique called *circular breathing* facilitates the flow of contracted energy and helps the breather release buried feelings. Circular breathing is performed by breathing freely and deeply in a continuous flow (with no pauses between the inhale and exhale) for an extended period of time.[14]

Alternate Nostril Breath Cycles

Throughout the day, our bodies move through alternating two-hour (approximately) cycles that are conducive to either rest or activity. In the active phase, the brain's left hemisphere (connected to the right side of the body) is dominant. In the passive phase, the brain's right hemisphere (connected to the left side of the body) is dominant. The precipitating factor for these cycles seems to be the breath. In the active phase the right nostril is more open; while the left nostril dominates during the passive phase. At any given time (presuming you don't have a respiratory blockage), you can tell which nostril is dominant simply by pressing your finger against one nostril to close it, breathing only through the opposite nostril, and then reversing the process to see which side is more open. When the right nostril is dominant, it's a good time for exercise, eating, and engaging in other active pursuits. Cycles of left nostril dominance are more appropriate for rest, meditation, and passive pursuits, as well as for drinking fluids. Normally the cycles switch every two hours or so, but occasionally (due to stress or depression) you can get stuck in one mode for several hours.

For times when you are in a passive phase and need to be active, or are in an active phase when you're trying to sleep, you can coax your body to switch cycles. Lying on your right side tends to close the right nostril and open the left one, so it's a good position for sleep or relaxation. Lying on your left side tends to have the opposite effect—it closes the left nostril and makes you feel more active. You also can manually close one nostril for a few seconds to encourage the opposite one to take over, breathe that way for a few seconds, and then release the nostril and breathe normally. Repeat this pattern several times until the desired nostril becomes dominant. Rather than forcibly shifting nostril dominance, however, it's best to honor your body's rhythms and match your activities to the existing cycle. Reserve methods of altering nostril dominance for times when you feel you've been in one mode for an extended period.

Challenges to Awareness

Preventing Procrastination

Each time you think about doing something but don't do it, you devote time and energy to the task without truly accomplishing anything. For instance, if a chair in your bedroom is piled with garments that need cleaning or mending, every time you see it you say to yourself, "I really should get those clothes taken care of." You carry this nagging thought with you, and it consumes some of your mental energy. The same applies to the broken appliance in the kitchen and the stack of unopened mail on the hall table.

The solution to ending this waste of mental energy is simple: do the jobs that are nagging at you. If it isn't practical to complete a task immediately, then schedule it on your calendar as you would any other appointment. For repetitive tasks, schedule a block of time every day, week, or month. With paying bills, for example, either deal with each bill immediately or schedule some time every week or two to handle the bills that have accumulated. Also, don't stop working when you have almost completed a job—a mostly-done task is still an undone task. Completing the job allows you to cross it off your list, both literally and figuratively.

The more obstacles that exist between you and an activity, the less likely you are to engage in that activity. For example, you join a health club and plan to work out there three times a week. Each time you want to exercise, you must change into the appropriate clothing, collect your workout gear, drive to the health club, sign in at the front desk, go to the locker room to store your gear, and get in line to wait for the equipment. All this, and you haven't even started to exercise yet!

This principle can be used to your advantage when trying to break a habit. To cut down on smoking, for instance, purchase no more than one pack of cigarettes at a time. You may find that when you want a cigarette, you don't want it badly enough to go to the trouble of getting your car keys and wallet, driving to the store, and standing in line.

Handling Habits

Most people have what I call *global characteristics*: patterns expressed in many diverse aspects of their lives. For instance, I tend to do things a little at a time. I sip water throughout the day, eat several snacks and small meals in lieu of two or three large meals, and pay bills promptly rather than waiting until they pile up. A friend of mine prefers to do things in batches: he drinks water infrequently but in large amounts, eats two meals a day, and pays bills twice a month. Global characteristics can be broad ranging and include traits such as perfectionism, impulsiveness, procrastination, overindulgence, thoroughness, and neatness.

There is a physical, electromagnetic reality to habits and patterns. It's even possible to take on other people's habits in the same way we tend to follow an existing path rather than creating our own path. It is easier to do something when someone else has done it before you, even if you aren't aware that they have. I realized the pervasiveness of habit patterns several years ago when an out-of-town friend visited me for a few days. In my house the bedrooms were upstairs, with the master bedroom on the left and the guest bedroom on the right. My friend was annoyed at herself because every time she climbed the stairs, she automatically turned left although she knew she should turn right. Finally we realized the cause of her seemingly illogical behavior: she was following the strong "energy path" to the master bedroom that was created not only by my partner and me, but also by the couple who had lived there before us.

The birds that frequent my backyard provided another demonstration of the tendency to follow old patterns. The little songbirds like to eat seeds from the hanging feeder, as do the larger birds. In their pursuit of the sunflower seeds mixed with millet and corn, the larger birds were scattering the songbird food on the ground. Also I noticed that the songbirds usually left the feeder when the larger birds arrived. I decided the best solution was to buy the songbirds a special feeder that was too small for the other birds to access. I kept the old feeder and filled it with sunflower seeds for the larger birds. This seemed to be an ideal setup—the songbirds would have their own feeder, and the other birds could have as many sunflower seeds as they wanted.

However, I soon observed that the songbirds did not use the new feeder but continued to frequent the old one, ferreting out the last of the songbird food from among the sunflower seeds. It was frustrating to watch them scrounging for the few little seeds left on the ground and in the old feeder, when the fully stocked songbird feeder was right next to it. To access this cornucopia, the songbirds had only to notice the new feeder and find the openings. Ultimately I resorted to drastic measures: I removed the old feeder and put the new feeder in exactly the same place. Finally the songbirds started using the new feeder. After allowing them to practice their new habit for a few days, I hung the old feeder on the other side of the pole for the larger birds.

It occurred to me that the songbirds were acting much like humans do—continuing to follow established patterns even when they no longer serve us. Tightly locked into our old habits, we fail to notice new opportunities that are right in front of us, ripe for the picking. All too often, we investigate these opportunities only when outside circumstances force us to change (when the old feeder is taken away, so to speak).

Trying to change an ingrained habit typically requires a period of almost constant vigilance. It reminds me of training a dog. You lead the animal away from something he's not supposed to be bothering, but as soon as you turn your attention away, the dog goes back to doing the very thing you just corrected him for! With persistence, eventually the new pattern takes hold.

4

Conscious Creation

o o o o o o o o o o o o o o o o o o o o o o o o o o o o o o o

"You create what you concentrate upon—not what you think, *for your concentration is not based in thought. Your concentration is based in your beliefs."*

—*Elias*[15]

Creating Our Own Reality

Introduced into popular culture by Jane Roberts's Seth books, the expression "you create your own reality" has become a New Age catchphrase.[16] Yet even those who follow these philosophies can find it hard to believe we create everything in our reality, nor do we understand how. Because we don't understand how we create, we ascribe creations we are pleased with to good luck or divine intervention. When something happens that we don't like, we attribute it to bad luck or punishment from some deity. Yet in every case, we are the creators of our own experience. There really is no such thing as luck, and no deity is directing the events of our day-to-day existence.

For most of my life, I believed there were two kinds of people: those who made things happen and those whom things happened to…and that I was clearly in the latter category. Eventually I discovered that this view was very distorted. In truth, each of us is responsible for creating everything in our experience. This includes, of course, our physical bodies and the way we experience aging. It is *all* under our control.

Energy Follows Attention

The axiom "energy flows where attention goes" is one I've found to be true. When we pay attention to something, we're putting our energy there, and energy is what causes physical manifestations and draws things into our experience. Following are two stories that illustrate how moving one's attention can result in tangible changes in areas that seem to be out of our control.

When mobile telephones first started becoming widely used (but notably, before I had one myself), sometimes I noticed cars being driven poorly because the driver's attention was focused on a phone conversation. After this happened a couple of times in quick succession, I began to get annoyed at just the idea of people talking on the phone while driving. Within a few weeks, I was encountering phone-using bad drivers several times a day. The more attention I paid to drivers talking on mobile phones, the worse the problem got. One day when I was trying to get to work expeditiously, I ended up on a two-lane road behind a large pickup truck traveling well below the posted speed limit. The driver was talking on a mobile phone and seemed distracted. He was having difficulty even staying in his own lane, so trying to pass him didn't seem like a good idea. After enduring this painfully slow trip, I decided I needed to do something about my growing problem with mobile phones and bad drivers. My solution was to force myself to stop noticing and judging drivers who were using phones. When I did notice such a driver, I reminded myself that the person had a right to talk on the phone while driving, and that it didn't have to affect me unless I allowed it to. After this attitude adjustment, I encountered fewer and fewer incidents of bad drivers using mobile phones. Soon it was no longer a problem for me.

Could my shift in attitude have affected the number of people who chose to use phones while driving, or did it cause people to drive more skillfully while talking on the phone? No, of course not. I create my own reality, not that of other people. Shifting my attention (and not focusing on my belief that talking on the phone while driving was irresponsible) resulted in a change in the type of experiences I drew to myself. It works this way with everything, which is why prejudice against a certain category of people can be so insidious. Someone with negative beliefs about a particular group will attract a disproportionate number of people from that group who fulfill his pessimistic expectations. These experiences serve to strengthen the belief, and it becomes a vicious circle.

The second example of how moving one's attention can result in actual, physical changes involves a plant. In the springtime my housemate and I bought a beautiful, bright pink bougainvillea that graced our backyard all summer. These plants do not take well to extreme cold, so when fall arrived we moved the bougainvillea indoors. Right away, I noticed it dropped so many leaves and petals onto the carpet that I could barely finish cleaning up one batch before more would appear. The bougainvillea's constant defoliating became an annoyance, and I wondered if it had been a mistake to buy the plant. Its shedding of leaves and petals seemed to increase every week. Then one day, after picking up a plethora leaves and petals from the carpet, I looked—really looked—at the plant instead of at the carpet beneath it. The bougainvillea was bursting with gorgeous pink blossoms! For weeks I had noticed only the dead leaves and petals and failed to even look at the plant itself. For the next few minutes, I drank in the beauty it offered, apologizing to the bougainvillea for having ignored it for so long. "With your beauty," I told the plant, "it's okay with me if you drop just as many leaves and petals as you want."

Later that day, I walked by the bougainvillea again. Typically it would have dropped at least a dozen leaves and petals in the amount of time since my last cleanup, but it hadn't lost a single one! In the days that followed, I noticed that the plant's defoliating decreased markedly. It wasn't just my imagination; my housemate commented on the change as well. I didn't move the bougainvillea, change its watering schedule, or do anything other than switch my attention from the dropped leaves and petals to the plant itself. When I paid attention to the dead foliage, I got more dead foliage. When I shifted my attention to the beauty of the plant, I got more beauty—the bougainvillea thrived. Think about *that* the next time you start counting gray hairs!

This experience can serve as a metaphor for what many of us do habitually: we pay attention to things that annoy us and put a lot of effort into dealing with them. The solution is not to spend more time and effort "cleaning up dead leaves." All we need to do is to move our attention from what we *don't* want to what we *do* want.

How Creation Works

We create our reality internally and project it outward, which is what creates our external world. Most of us tend to focus on the external reality almost exclusively. It's as if we are looking in a mirror observing the reflection of ourselves and what we're generating, but we're paying attention only to the reflection and forgetting what (and who) is creating it. It's like a man looking in the mirror and noticing that his hair is in an unflattering style, his face is covered with stubble, and his tie is askew. Rather than changing his hairstyle, shaving his face, and straightening his tie, he tries to alter the reflection by sheer force of will. He has an idea of the improvements he'd like to make, but instead of taking action that would change himself (and therefore the image he's projecting), he focuses positive energy at his reflection and appeals to nonphysical sources for help in altering the reflection. Of course, nothing really changes.

Most us tend not to pay attention to the feelings, thoughts, and beliefs that can reveal what we are creating internally. Instead we scramble around, engaging in action that gets us nowhere. I've noticed that when I easily create something I want, often I didn't really *do* anything except get out of my own way. In many cases, if I had stopped to ruminate on the matter, I probably would have short-circuited what turned out to be an effortless creation. The key to effective, purposeful creating is simply to *allow it to happen* rather than analyzing all the things we are doing wrong and trying to correct them.

Another ineffective strategy (or lack of strategy) is sitting around and waiting for something to happen, which seems to be the bane of many spiritually-oriented people. It's far more productive to focus on ideas and formulate them into tangible creations rather than waiting for something nebulous to fall out of the sky. When we have an intention and truly expect it to be fulfilled, it usually is. Expecting your desire to be fulfilled, however, doesn't mean you won't have to take any action. At times you will be inspired to take action; follow these impulses even if they don't seem to make sense at first. Often you'll find that things will fall into place without any great effort or frenetic activity on your part.

From Concept to Creation

When you have an idea for a creation that obviously requires physical action to manifest (such as a new business or a house), it's helpful to take a structured approach. Here is a basic framework that can be applied to almost any endeavor:

1. Initiate the idea.
2. Define and give structure to the idea.
3. Formulate plans for carrying out the idea.
4. Follow the plans, taking any action required.

This approach is different from taking action aimlessly; the physical actions are accomplished in the final step of the process. It's common for people to get stuck in the first two steps and just stay there. Conversely, sometimes we try to go from step 1 directly to step 4, which doesn't work either. As a general rule, it's important to follow the steps in order.

Focus Areas

When clarifying general intentions (such as those related to improvements in health or appearance), it's unwise to set deadlines for their manifestation. The concept of a *deadline* is limiting; even the word itself has negative connotations. The term *goal* is more positive but still connotes completion at a certain point, which isn't always appropriate. *Focus area* is the expression I like best. People excel in the areas where they focus their attention and energy. Individuals who are outstanding in a particular field are those who concentrate most intensely on that subject or activity. This is true not only of geniuses, but of so-called idiot savants—they tune out distractions and focus with extreme intensity on the task at hand. Our culture teaches us to scatter our energies, provides constant distractions, and places a high value on multitasking. Many of us lose touch at an early age with our inherent ability to concentrate.

Impediments to Creation

In theory, to get what we want, we simply need to make a choice, set an intention, and then allow it to manifest. In practice, this often isn't as easy as it sounds. In Jane Roberts's book *The Nature of Personal Reality*, Seth (the famous nonphysical personality) stated, "You get what you concentrate upon. There is no other main rule."[17] Many people have misinterpreted this statement to mean you get what you think about, which isn't necessarily the case. Concentration involves your beliefs and intentions, not simply your thoughts. Following are a few of the reasons why we have difficulty manifesting what we want.

Indecision

In situations where you feel you can't make a decision and are continually vacillating, your indecision stalls the creation process. Ensuring that you make the best choice is often less important than the action of making *some* choice. By making a choice, you put your energy fully behind that choice instead of dissipating it by ruminating over the various alternatives. If it turns out that the choice doesn't serve your intentions very well, then you can make another choice in the future. We always have options, even if we don't recognize them right away.

A good example of the downside of indecision is an employee who is dissatisfied with her job and can't decide whether to stay or find a new one. Due to her uncertainty, she isn't fully present in the job and doesn't perform it as well as she could. Her half-hearted attempts at looking for other employment opportunities don't yield substantial results either. In cases like this, what often happens is that eventually an (apparently) external event forces the person into action. The company will reorganize or downsize, and the employee (who probably was not one of the top performers) will be let go. Ultimately she will find another job, but it would have been more advantageous for her to look for new employment on her own schedule, before she really needed it. If she had made the decision to stay in her current job, her performance probably would have been better, and it's possible the company would have retained her as an employee.

At times when you feel you cannot make a decision or accomplish something you need to do, try substituting the word *won't* for *can't*. "I won't make a decision" has a very different meaning than, "I can't make a decision." When we say we won't do something, it connotes a choice rather than an inability. This simple change of semantics alters our perception and helps us recognize that the power is in our own hands.

Another helpful approach is to substitute the word *choice* for *decision*. *Decision* is a serious word that connotes restriction and finality. *Choice* sounds more light-hearted and appealing; it seems less permanent and more open to future possibilities. Think about the ways we typically use these words: We must *decide* which job to take or college to attend, while we *choose* a flavor of ice cream or the color of a new shirt.

Conflicting Beliefs

Our world is based upon beliefs—virtually everything we think is a truth is actually a belief. Beliefs themselves are neither good nor bad, but a certain belief may be inappropriate for a particular individual. If you align with a belief or set of beliefs, then you are bound by its rules and limitations. If you don't align with it, then those rules don't affect you. It's as simple as that. The difficulty arises when we hold two or more beliefs that conflict with each other.

Regarding aging, our culture has two strong beliefs that are completely incompatible. The first is that youth is highly desirable and any evidence of aging is undesirable. The second is that age-related degeneration is natural and largely unavoidable. A person who holds both of these beliefs is obviously going to have problems. If you align with only one of them, you're far less likely to experience conflict about aging (and probably wouldn't be reading this book!). Most of us align with both beliefs, at least to some degree; therefore we experience conflict about getting older.

Some people choose not to buy into the first belief (that youth is good and aging is bad). In what is often called "aging gracefully," they accept the changes they believe are an inevitable part of growing older—without feeling discontented and losing self-esteem. In this book, I'm obviously addressing the second belief (that age-related degeneration is natural and unavoidable). Neither approach is superior; it's simply a preference.

Unfortunately, many of our beliefs are so ingrained that they're transparent to us—we don't even realize they are beliefs. A good way to recognize your beliefs is to make a point of noticing your automatic reactions, feelings, and thoughts. Behind each of these is a belief (often multiple beliefs). For at least one day, carry paper with you and make note of all the beliefs you are able to identify.

Here is a strategy for dealing with conflicting beliefs:

1. Notice your automatic reactions—how you feel and what you think, say, and do.
2. Identify the beliefs that underlie these reactions and choices.
3. Remind yourself that they are beliefs, not unalterable truths.
4. Recognize the areas in which you have conflicting beliefs.
5. Offer yourself a choice as to which beliefs you want to align with.

Sometimes our beliefs about what we want are inconsistent with our beliefs about what is possible for us. If we don't believe it is probable (or even possible) that we can manifest something, then it's unlikely we will. Conscious creating is a continuum: doubt, hope, expectation, certainty. The closer you are to certainty, the greater the likelihood that what you want will manifest. Contrary to a popular New Age principle, we do not create through our thoughts. You can think positive thoughts until the cows come home, but the cows *won't* come home unless you truly believe they will.

Focusing on Lack

When we want something (health, a youthful appearance, money, or a happy relationship), we often focus more on the lack of it than on having it. We attract what we focus upon, so when we focus on lack, we get more lack. This is a common reason for not manifesting what we desire. Sick people who concentrate on their disease will get more disease. Individuals who focus on their shortage of money will continue to manifest a shortage. Those who have experienced trauma and keep thinking and/or talking about the experience (including in a support group setting) are likely to continue to feel the effects of the trauma. If they focus on it enough, they may even attract similar experiences in the future.

Focusing on lack can also be done collectively, which often happens when there are drought conditions in an area. People start focusing on the lack of rain, so that's precisely what they get: more lack of rain. A more productive way to think about a drought is that it's similar to when a person goes on a crash diet—he can keep it up for a while, but eventually he binges. That's what a geographical area does when there's a drought: it goes on a moisture starvation diet, which is unnatural. Ultimately it reverts back to its natural state and rains. Once it starts raining, it often rains a lot, just like a person who abandons a strict diet and goes on an eating spree. This is nature's way of keeping a balance.

A couple of years ago in the area where I live, weather conditions had been unusually dry for a long time. A common topic of conversation was the drought: how bad it was getting, the likelihood of increased water restrictions, and the dire consequences that could occur if the drought continued. With the intention to do something constructive about the situation, several friends and I pooled our energies. We stated our intention for rain, visualizing and imagining how it would be when it was raining. I thought of the rainy spring and summer days we used to have in Virginia when I was a child—how the rain felt and smelled, what it looked and sounded like, and how much fun it was to play in the mud puddles afterward. Other group members started talking about what it was like for them during a rain shower. Two days later, it rained for the first time in weeks—a steady, soaking rain that lasted many hours. During the next few days, it rained periodically.

In our culture, we have been taught to solve problems by focusing on them (the conventional medical system is based on this premise), and learning not to do so can seem daunting. To change the habit of focusing on problems, you must first be aware that you are doing it. To catch yourself when you start concentrating on the negative, pay attention to your, feelings, thoughts, words, and actions. If you find it difficult to keep your attention on the positive (health instead of illness, for example), then switch focus and change the subject completely. Stop thinking about health or finances and start thinking about your favorite vacation area or your cat. Put on some music that will lift your mood, start reading that new novel, or play hide-and-seek with your kids. Improving your mood and attitude makes a difference in the type of experiences you attract—including those that seem to be completely out of your control. Even if it has no discernable effect on your experiences, at least you'll feel better.

Attachment to the Outcome

Think of a beam lying on the floor. If you want to walk across the length of the beam without falling off, you probably can do so without much difficulty. Now visualize the same beam suspended above a 50-meter chasm. Could you walk across the beam with the same ease you did before? Probably not. But it's the same beam, so what's the difference? The difference is *attachment to the outcome.* When the beam was on the floor, you were willing to walk across it and accept the outcome whether you stayed on or fell off. With the beam higher up, however, you would be unwilling to accept the outcome of falling off, which likely would result in serious injury or death. It's the same with most things in life—if we are not attached to the outcome, we can accomplish them almost effortlessly. It is our attachment to the outcome that causes us to contract in fear and restrict the natural flow that allows us to fulfill our intentions with ease.

When deciding whether to go into a new business, I gave a lot of thought to what it takes to achieve business success—how to identify a good opportunity, why some people succeed and others fail, and so forth. I'd met several people who had done well in that business, and I looked for a common denominator among them. I discovered that when most of them started, they were not a position where they truly needed the money. They weren't coming from a place of lack and were not attached to the outcome. In contrast, people who borrow money to invest in a business must be attached to the outcome because they have to pay back the investors. The ones who succeed anyway tend to be those with a strong belief in both their own capabilities and the value of their business.

In the same vein, I noticed that with job interviews, if I really wanted a particular position, I usually wouldn't receive an offer. Yet if I had a "take it or leave it" attitude about the job, the employer often did make an offer. When I desperately wanted the position, my attachment to the outcome short-circuited its manifestation.

Flexibility (not being attached to a specific result) is also a great help in conscious creation. As long as it doesn't conflict with your life intentions, you can have virtually anything you want if you're flexible about how it manifests. For example, a college student who needs a reliable car but doesn't have the financial resources to buy one should not limit himself to wanting only a vehicle of a particular make, model, color, and year. It may turn out that a relative is planning to trade in her stylish, well-maintained car for a larger vehicle, and she would be happy to sell the car to the student for a modest sum. When specifying your desires, be as flexible as possible while still being happy with the potential result.

Perfectionism

If you are trying to be perfect, your fear of making mistakes can inhibit your desire to take action, leading to a state of inertia and stagnation. Striving for perfection also results in inflexibility and an unwillingness to try new things. "Mistakes" are simply learning experiences we choose to label in a negative way. Rather than striving for perfection, aim for improvement. Perfection is a paradox: nothing is ever really perfect, yet everything is perfect just as it is. Perfection implies completeness, and everything is in a continuous state of becoming. In the objective sense, perfection is an unreachable goal. Do the best you can and just go with it. Even if you find fault with the result, it may turn out later that you like the actual outcome better than the one you thought you wanted.

Although we characterize virtually everything as either good or bad, there really are no good or bad decisions; we just choose different experiences. The greatest regrets in life are not the things you've done that didn't work out well—they are the things you wanted to do but didn't have the courage, energy, or self-confidence to pursue.

Intention Versus Wants

There is a difference between *intention* and *wants*. Our emotions may indicate we want something, but if having it does not support our fundamental life intentions (the life plan of our inner self), then it's unlikely the desire will be manifested. I may want a particular job, for instance, but having that job may not support the intention of my inner self—an intention I may not be paying attention to consciously. In cases where I seem to do everything right (and don't have conflicting beliefs blocking the manifestation) but it doesn't work, I usually conclude that what I want would not be appropriate for me at that time.

Most of us assume we are aware of our intentions, but this isn't always the case. For instance, nearly everyone says they would like to win the lottery, but actually having it happen would be disturbing to most people. Their way of life would change abruptly; they would be forced out of their comfort zone and subjected to media attention and demands from family, friends, and strangers. They would have to decide how to invest and/or spend the money, and they might feel guilty for not using it to help those in need. The surefire way to avoid these pressures and choices is to *not* win the lottery…so most of us don't.

Resentment

When we have struggled with something and then observe someone who achieved the same or better results without the struggle, it's natural to feel some resentment. Not only are we likely to envy the person, we also may feel their experience somehow invalidates our own achievement—or our pain. If we slaved for years to reach a goal and then discover that another person reached or exceeded the same goal in less time and with less effort, we feel as if our time and effort were wasted. In fact, nothing was wasted; we choose to experience things (yes, it's a choice) for the value of the experience, not simply as a means to an end. I've noticed that when I have something I think other people might envy, I tend to either discount it in some way or make a point of how hard I worked for it. Feeling I must justify my success or "good fortune" is aligning with limiting beliefs as well.

Each of us has areas in which things come easily and other areas we find challenging. Rather than resenting those who find our difficult areas easy, we can consider them examples of what is possible. As long as we begrudge others having money, business success, good health, beauty, a fulfilling relationship, or anything else we covet, we won't be able to create it for ourselves. *You cannot become what you resent.*

Creating Wealth

Money (or in New Age parlance, *abundance*) is a subject intrinsically related to how we experience life. Like emotional baggage and physical clutter, financial worries can affect how a person experiences aging. Some of the most common limiting beliefs about money are that money is scarce and hard to acquire, having money isn't spiritual, making a lot of money means you've "sold out," and wealth leads to unhappiness.

It's common for even middle-class people to have a "poverty mentality." They make enough money to cover their basic expenses and are not in serious debt, yet they worry about every expenditure, hold on tightly to material things in general, and resent those who have more than they do. Because they restrict the natural flow of resources, their income is low. In contrast, people who have an abundance mentality tend to draw opportunities—and to recognize and act on these opportunities. Those with a poverty mentality are less likely to attract opportunities, and they rarely take advantage of those that do come their way.

People who worry about money a great deal and fret over virtually every expenditure seem to have difficulty acquiring wealth. Often they work hard but have little to show for their efforts. I've experienced this myself. Several years ago when I moved to a new city and had trouble getting a job, I became very thrifty and worried about even small purchases. And what did this frugality get me? A job where I worked hard, contributed significantly to the company, and regularly participated in management meetings—yet was paid a low salary with no benefits. In sharp contrast are the people who have the attitude that money is plentiful and easy to make. They don't become stressed about finances and seem to attract wealth almost effortlessly.

If we could think of money the way we think of air, we wouldn't experience scarcity. Air is more essential to our physical survival than food, water, or anything else money can buy. If deprived of oxygen for more than a few minutes, we perish. Yet most of us never worry about getting enough air. We have no doubt that the next time we need to take a breath, there will be plenty of oxygen—and there always is. If we had the same limiting beliefs about air that most of us have about money, we would try to breathe in as much air as possible and hold it in as long as we could. People would live in fear that there wouldn't be enough air for everyone, resenting those who seemed to use more than their fair share of this invisible elixir. Hoarding air in storage tanks would be commonplace, and people would write their wills with a provision to leave the storage tanks to their loved ones. This scenario may sound ridiculous, but it's no more ridiculous than our insecurity about the availability of money or other material resources. It is our belief in scarcity (based upon lack of trust in ourselves) that creates conditions of insufficient resources.

Body Consciousness

One of the keys to establishing communication and cooperation with a life form is to recognize and appreciate its attributes. Our physical bodies are made up of a variety of conscious "beings" such as organs and cells. Most of us take for granted the functions they perform well, but if there's a problem, we get angry at the offending body part.

What if, instead of noticing only the things we don't like, we acknowledged some of the innumerable ways in which our bodies serve us very well? For instance, rather than becoming angry at your skin over a pimple or rash, think of all the beneficial things your skin does for you: it protects your body, helps insulate and cool you, allows you to feel the pleasure of touch, and gives you an attractive appearance. Getting angry at your skin for a small problem is like being an unappreciative boss with an excellent, hard-working employee. The employee puts in many hours and does a superb job without needing any supervision, yet the boss never notices. If, however, the employee does something the boss disapproves of, the boss reads him the riot act. The employee very likely will conclude that the boss doesn't notice or care about all his hard work, and he may lose motivation.

If we develop communication and cooperation with all aspects of our body, then we can facilitate its functioning and more easily determine the cause of any problems that occur. Instead of looking at yourself and noticing only what you think needs improvement, start focusing on the traits you like. If you observe something that seems out of place, ask your body to let you know what the problem is and what you can do to help. Clear your mind and allow the communication to come through. Very likely (although perhaps not immediately), you will receive information that gives you insight into the cause of the problem and what you can do to help your body restore its balance.

Manifesting Physical Changes

A young man I know was distressed that he was losing hair at a rapid rate. To make matters worse, he had been advised that his type of hair loss did not respond well to pharmaceutical oral or topical treatments. His problem was interesting to me because it was analogous to challenges most of us have experienced with physical conditions and characteristics we want to change. It seems that the more we resist the undesirable manifestation, the worse it gets. After pondering my friend's difficulty, a thought came into my mind: *You must accept your creation before you can make another choice.* I'd heard this idea before in different terms, and it seemed to have validity. I started thinking of a method to reach this state of acceptance, and came up with the following ideas.

The first step is to develop the attitude of feeling neutral about the condition or characteristic. You might not be happy about it, but you aren't resisting it either. When you are truly in a state of acceptance (nonresistance), you can choose to alter the physical manifestation—or not. The primary challenge, of course, is how to arrive at this state of acceptance. When I was younger, I used to be extremely critical about many of my physical features. One thing that helped was noticing people I admired who had similar characteristics: models, actresses, and women I'd met personally. When I noticed that a person I thought was attractive possessed some of the same traits I did, it made it easier to accept those traits in myself.

For my friend who was concerned about impending baldness, I suggested he talk with men who obviously had been bald for a number of years and seemed comfortable with their appearance. It's likely they would remember how it felt when they started losing their hair, and they probably would be open to sharing their experiences and perspective with him. I also suggested he discuss the subject with female friends. When the topic has come up with women I know, most have said they find bald men just as attractive as those with a full head of hair.

For the second step of the method—making another choice—it is necessary to believe you *can* make a different choice. It helps to read accounts of people who have made drastic physical changes believed by medical science to be impossible. *The Holographic Universe* includes quite a few of these stories, and they're well documented. In one case, it shows the before-and-after X-rays of a man who regenerated his hipbones after they had been destroyed by arthritis.[18] If someone can actually grow new hipbones, I told my friend, it shouldn't be too hard to grow hair! There are about 100,000 hair follicles on the scalp, many of which are dormant most of the time and can be activated.

Another key factor for manifesting physical changes is to *stop paying attention to what you don't like.* When we focus on something we don't like, we continually recreate it in each moment. To deal with a hair loss issue, for example, stop paying attention to your hairline, how much hair is falling out, and so forth. When you look in the mirror, probably the first thing you notice is your hairline. Catch yourself having this automatic reaction and switch your focus to another feature, preferably one you like—anything but your hair and hairline. At first you may have to force yourself to do this, but soon it will become a habit. If you notice a lot of hair on your pillow or in your comb, remind yourself that it's just old hairs falling out to make way for new ones. Trust yourself to create whatever will best serve your intentions.

Visualization

Visualization practices can sometimes be helpful for understanding the dynamics that are creating a physical condition, as well as for making changes. The following visualization technique is simple and can easily be tailored to your own preferences.

When you are ready to begin your visualization, if you aren't already in a positive, optimistic mood, do whatever will get you into this state. Listen to music, read something inspirational, play with your pet, or walk by a flower garden. Relax your body and clear your mind. It often helps to spend a few minutes in a meditative state before starting the visualization process.

Visualization includes not only mental images (which some people find difficult to create), but feelings, sensations, sounds, and scents. As much as possible, imagine yourself truly experiencing what you want your future to be like. It's essential to make this state feel authentic, so you may want to start small rather than reaching for the sky. For instance, if you have a long-term weight problem, you may not yet be able to envision yourself as very slender, but you probably can imagine comfortably wearing clothes a few sizes smaller than you wear now. Continue your visualization only as long as it holds your interest and makes you feel good—probably five minutes at most. If you start having contradictory feelings or thoughts ("I could never look that way"), then it's time to end the exercise. The images and feelings you generate in the visualization are themselves a creation, one you can tap into at any time throughout the day. Even momentary flashes of your internal creation will help it manifest in the physical world.

A slightly different type of visualization technique can be used to create a specific bodily condition. This method is particularly effective with health and appearance-related concerns. Here is an example of using this type of visualization to stimulate hair growth: Imagine a field of wheat in which some of the plants are green and supple while others are old and dry (coarse, gray hairs). Perhaps the ground (scalp) is dry and cracked; there may be bare (bald) patches where no plants are growing. Imagine the ground becoming rehydrated (improved circulation), new plants sprouting in the bare patches, and old stalks becoming green and supple (coarse, gray hairs regaining their original color and texture). Once you have developed this visualization, you can refer to it whenever you think of your hair and scalp, reminding yourself of the changes being made.

5

Emotional Clearing

○ ○

"Paradise is there, behind that door, in the next room, but I have lost the key. Perhaps I have only mislaid it."

—Kahlil Gibran

Self-Acceptance

The lack of self-acceptance (along with its companion, lack of self-trust) is fundamental to most of the problems we experience in our lives. Paradoxically, accepting ourselves as we are now (not as we expect to be after we've increased our income, lost weight, or met the right partner) not only allows us to be happier in the moment, it helps attract the things we desire. After all, if we feel we won't be "good enough" until we have these things, then we probably don't feel we're good enough to deserve them. It can become a vicious circle that leaves us chronically unhappy and dissatisfied.

There probably are only about half a dozen people in the world who fully accept themselves, and I doubt I've ever met one. In all seriousness, it seems that virtually everyone feels he or she is deficient in some manner. It's easy to understand how those with major physical or mental challenges could feel this way; it can be difficult to maintain self-esteem when immersed in a culture with belief systems that rate a person's worth on arbitrary standards you know you don't match. Yet haven't you ever looked at yourself as objectively as possible and concluded that you must be nuts to be so full of self-doubt? It's the feeling you get when you're walking down the street, feeling inadequate because you gained a little weight, got a B instead of an A on a test, or didn't make that tough sale. Then you see a disabled person who has to put forth major effort just to propel himself a short distance down the street. What do most of us really have to complain about? Sometimes I imagine us after we've passed on from this world, looking back on our lives and feeling like fools because we wasted so much time and energy worrying about what was "wrong" with us.

A couple of years ago, I began to pay close attention to what I said to people. I noticed that often my intention was to convince others or myself that I was not deficient or at fault in some way. It was disconcerting to discover that, rather than constructively addressing the issue at hand, I was starting out from the premise that I had to justify myself or prove my adequacy. Unfortunately, this mode of operation is quite common; I've noticed that many people do the same thing. It would be much more productive if we started from a premise of adequacy and focused our energy on our creations.

The best way I've found to get out of the mode of doubting myself is to develop the habit of paying attention to what I'm doing, thinking, and feeling in the moment. Focusing my attention in this manner interrupts the pattern of projecting my self-judgment onto other people. (In fact, they're probably too busy judging themselves to worry about me!) This recommendation has been given by numerous self-help and metaphysical sources, yet it was the one thing I really wanted to avoid. Paying attention to what is going on inside myself is a lot like looking in the mirror on a bad hair day—I'd rather pay attention to almost anything else. Yet we create our reality from the inside out, so self-awareness is fundamental to conscious creation.

Mirroring

Everything in our outside environment is a manifestation of what is inside us. If we fail to recognize our own characteristics, we will see them mirrored in the people and events around us, sometimes in an exaggerated fashion. Erin, for example, thought she had come to terms with her unhappy childhood, but deep down she still felt bitter over her absent father and lack of parental support. Intellectually, she understood that her parents had done the best they could under the circumstances, but emotionally, she still held resentment. Then she became romantically involved with a newly divorced man who had a daughter close to the age Erin had been when her parents separated. Despite Erin's attempts to befriend her, the girl was surly and resentful. After months of frustration over the situation, Erin realized she had drawn it into her experience due to her own unacknowledged childhood issues. Her boyfriend's daughter was reflecting Erin's own deeply held resentments. This realization made it easier for her to deal with the daughter's hostility; she understood that in a way, the girl was "acting out" for both of them. Eventually the resentment abated and they become friends.

The mirroring concept also applies in *feng shui* (the Chinese art of placement), which has become popular in the past few years. When a person has problems with finances, for example, it isn't because the prosperity areas in his home are poorly arranged. It's the other way around: the arrangement of the prosperity areas reflects the way he handles his finances. People design their environment in a way that mirrors their beliefs, and the environment reinforces those beliefs. Feng shui techniques often work because the person recognizes her beliefs, realizes they don't serve her, and alters her physical surroundings to reflect her new attitudes. The external changes may help her avoid slipping back into old patterns. It's also possible to jump-start inner changes by making physical alterations. Anything from getting a massage to cleaning out a closet can lead to seemingly unrelated life changes.

Judgment and Negativity

Right and wrong are simply a matter of perspective. Virtually everyone acts out of good intentions—what they believe to be for the higher good—regardless of how terrible you may perceive their actions to be. Judgment is a natural product of holding beliefs, and beliefs are inherent to our world. Telling yourself not to judge is a lot like telling yourself not to breathe: it's only a matter of time until you can't help but do it again. Judgment also involves choice, and it's important to distinguish between making choices for you (which is necessary and appropriate) and making choices for other people, which in most cases is inappropriate. When making choices for yourself, think of it as *discernment* or *evaluation* rather than rather than judgment, which almost by definition incorporates negativity.

To minimize the amount of time and energy you spend in judgment about other people, get in the habit of remaining neutral rather than labeling things as positive or negative. *Neutrality* in this context means detachment, which is not the same as indifference. Indifference indicates a lack of caring, but you can be neutral and still feel concerned. When you can't help but go into judgment, simply observe your reactions in a detached way, without trying to suppress or intensify them.

Managing Negativity

If you are having negative feelings about something, try using a three-step method I call the Triple-A process (Acknowledge, Address, and Abandon):

1. *Acknowledge* what you are feeling; don't try to rationalize or deny it. Feelings are a form of communication. Overriding feelings with thoughts is like pushing a floating cork under the water—it's only a matter of time before it pops up again.

2. *Address* the issue or concern as best you can. Addressing the issue may involve taking action or simply venting your frustration by writing about it or doing some physical exercise. If you can't come up with an appropriate action, you may be able to address the issue by altering the way you think about it.

3. *Abandon* your thoughts about the issue—let it go and don't keep dwelling on it. At this point (in contradiction to the earlier example), you may have to push down the cork a few times until it gets waterlogged and stays down. If you find you still keep thinking about the issue, then it's likely you haven't adequately addressed it yet.

An even simpler technique for dealing with negativity is to honestly assess what, if any, benefit there is to having the negative thoughts and judgments. What is the worst that could happen if you didn't have these thoughts? Is there anything constructive you can do about the situation that you aren't doing (or haven't done) already? Imagine how you would feel if you stopped having the negative thoughts and judgments—would you feel better or worse than you do now? Consider how differently you might treat other people (and yourself) if you weren't judging them or you. If your imagined scenario seems like a happier one (and it almost always does), then you may find yourself choosing that alternative rather than continuing on your current track. When the judgments and negative thoughts are reframed as a conscious choice, it becomes obvious that the best option is the alternative that feels better. Don't try to force it; simply allow yourself to make a new choice.

Attaining Acceptance

In addition to understanding that age-related degeneration is not inevitable, an essential key to the aging dilemma is to *accept what you have already created*. That is, to acknowledge—without judgment—the health or appearance changes that are physical manifestations of a belief in degeneration. Acceptance does not mean you have to like these conditions, nor does it mean you can't change them. Paradoxically, truly accepting what you have created is what allows you to make a different choice. It's perfectly okay to use health therapies, cosmetic treatments, or other physical means of improving the functioning or appearance of something that isn't to your liking. Knowing you have these options can make it easier to accept a condition you find uncomfortable or unappealing. It is quite possible, however, to alter these conditions without using physical methods. (Notice I used the word *condition* rather than *feature* or *characteristic*, which imply permanence.)

The concept of acceptance is paradoxical, which makes it difficult to explain in a way that makes logical sense. Accepting a condition does not mean you will be stuck with it for life. On the contrary, it gives you the freedom to make another choice. However, trying to accept something only because you want to change it is not true acceptance; it's just fooling yourself. True acceptance entails feeling okay about whatever you create: stiff joints or flexibility, baldness or a full head of hair, a slim figure or a portly one. Admittedly, this is much easier said than done. An additional challenge is that acceptance isn't necessarily permanent. You may be in a state of acceptance today, but tomorrow you might wake up feeling troubled by the same old issues. If this happens to you, hang in there. Every moment you spend in acceptance "counts" and makes it easier to sustain that state for longer periods. When I've reached a state of acceptance about aging issues, it's been very liberating.

For most of the time I was working on this book, the thought of speaking in public about aging made me very apprehensive. Although I am deeply inspired to share my knowledge on this subject with others, I was concerned that I might be criticized for not looking like a 25-year-old. (The irony is that I didn't look 25 even when I was 25! From my twenties to mid-thirties, people typically thought I was at least five years older than my actual age.) Since I understand that age-related degeneration is due to beliefs, I judged myself harshly for having some physical signs of aging. After all, I "know better," and therefore shouldn't be manifesting something I find undesirable.

Unfortunately, that isn't quite the way it works. Understanding these concepts on an intellectual level does not necessarily change one's limiting beliefs, at least not right away. My current beliefs are such that I'm quite confident about maintaining good health and optimum physical and mental functioning, but less confident about completely avoiding various aesthetic aspects of aging. Finally I acknowledged that it's okay for me not to be perfect; it doesn't invalidate the truth of the concepts. Putting pressure on oneself to look younger (and being attached to the outcome) just makes it more difficult to transcend limiting beliefs about aging.

Accepting What Is

Since it affects everything in our lives, addressing the lack of acceptance (of both ourselves and others) is well worth the effort. The challenge, of course, is finding a way to reach a state of acceptance regarding something you don't like. When you have thoughts like, "I weigh too much" or "I shouldn't have these lines around my eyes," question yourself. Why should or shouldn't you have the weight or wrinkles? In fact, you *do* have them; there's no "should" about it. They are part of you, something you've manifested. These conditions may not be what you prefer, but they aren't "bad." Ask yourself what is really wrong with having them—does it make you an unworthy person? It's doubtful that you consider other people with a full figure or facial lines to be unworthy, so there's no reason to judge yourself that way. There is nothing inherently wrong with any physical condition. Truly giving yourself permission to be the way you are is incredibly freeing. Following is an example of an insight I had recently that has made me more accepting of something I dislike about myself.

When I was 20 years old, I decided to get my brown hair frosted. The procedure consisted of donning a tight plastic cap with little holes in it, through which my hairstylist pulled strands of hair with what resembled a knitting needle. The strands were coated with a peroxide-containing emulsion, and then I sat under a hot hairdryer while it processed. The whole ordeal required about three hours and a sizeable chunk of my weekly paycheck.

I now prefer a more natural look and simply have my brown hair lightened a shade, which also covers the gray. Recently I looked in the mirror at my silver-streaked roots and thought, "Wow, I have frosted hair!" Ironically, it doesn't appear much different from the look I sought when I was 20. I don't particularly want frosted hair now (in truth, I looked a bit like a skunk when I left the salon that day), but it made me realize how silly it is to consider gray hair "bad" and frosted hair "good"—they're basically the same thing.

Another helpful approach for accepting physical conditions is to remind yourself that most of them are—or can be—temporary rather than permanent. This applies not only to conditions commonly believed to be easily changeable (such as body weight and muscle tone), but also to facial lines, thinning hair, and most health problems. There is virtually nothing about ourselves that we can't change. We create a "new" body in each moment—physical conditions appear permanent simply because we keep recreating them in the same way. Whenever you notice something about yourself (aesthetic or functional) that you dislike, remind yourself that it's temporary condition you can change—with or without using physical methods. In most cases, I find it easier to accept something undesirable if I believe it isn't permanent.

Clearing the Past

Unresolved emotional issues (often referred to as *emotional baggage*) can cause a person to feel old, which leads to age-related degeneration. Many people actually associate their wrinkles and gray hair with difficulties they have experienced. They wear them almost as a badge of accomplishment, like a battle-scarred veteran proud of his war wounds. Others would very much like to unload their emotional baggage, but fear they'll be stuck with it for life. If this is the case with you, don't give up—there are methods that can help.

A longstanding emotional issue such as long-term guilt or a traumatic memory is held in your energy field, and it affects you much like chewing gum stuck to your shoe. It is a constant, low-level annoyance that keeps you from moving efficiently. The more you walk, the more junk gets stuck to the gum, until eventually it seriously impedes your progress. The obvious solution is to remove the gum and all the attached debris. Sometimes you have to dislodge a lot of debris before you can even see the chewing gum (original problem) itself.

As best you can, jettison the past—wipe the slate clean of any resentment, bitterness, or grudges you are holding. Choose not to give attention to anything you have experienced that makes you feel bad when you think about it. There's no point in expending energy resenting what happened in the past, no matter how difficult or traumatic it may have been. The energy you put into resentment and ruminations about past injustices won't help you get over them; it may actually draw more such experiences to you in the future. It can be helpful to know what our fears and insecurities may stem from, but it's no excuse to keep recreating them in the present.

Victim mentality is the belief that something can be foisted upon you by another person or an outside force—that something can happen to you without your having a choice in the matter. You always have a choice, although you may not be consciously aware that you chose a "negative" experience. How one reacts to the resulting situation is irrelevant. A person who fights back can have victim mentality just as much as one who withdraws and feels sorry for himself. Rather than seeing myself as a victim, I now view past traumas and dramas as if everyone simply played out his or her role, like in the theater. Some people play the part of the bad guy and others play the victim, but everyone involved has agreed to participate. Viewing experiences in this manner helps me maintain a more neutral, nonjudgmental mind-set, removing the emotional charge from potentially distressing memories.

An alternative to working through emotional issues is to turn your attention and choose to focus on something else. If you truly can do this, it's the most efficient method for dealing with upsetting situations. Turning your attention is not the same as denying or burying feelings, although these actions can appear the same on the surface. If you cannot genuinely turn your attention to something else, then it's better to process and work through the feelings rather than trying to ignore them and pretending they don't exist. Inevitably, they'll surface later in some other form—possibly illness, depression, or anger over another issue. When you have negative feelings about something, forcing yourself to focus only on the positive aspects is a form of resistance—you are denying and resisting what *is*. Instead, accept the situation (with the realization that you've created it), feel the negative emotions, and let them flow through you like a boat's wake in the water. Don't erect a dam and try to pay attention only to what is on the calm side of the dam.

Resistance to Change

When people have chronic or long-term physical, emotional, or financial problems, their ego structure (which instinctively fears annihilation) tends to incorporate the characteristic as part of itself, almost like a vital organ or a limb. The ego then fights to keep the problem, no matter how miserable it's making the person. If the individual's self-image doesn't change, then the problem will remain, regardless of any treatment he receives. If a treatment is likely to work, he may reject it out of hand. At times, the ego-self needs to be treated like a stubborn, fearful dog that becomes aggressive when it perceives a threat. It's only trying to protect you, but it often perceives danger where there is none. The dog needs to be gently led; trying to force it will only make things worse. Sometimes I feel like telling my ego-self to go sit in a corner and chew on a bone, but just like a dog, it doesn't like being ignored and will bark until I pay attention to it.

It's helpful to evaluate your motives on a regular basis. Are you doing—or not doing—something out of fear (the need to avoid a negative consequence) or joy (the desire to manifest something positive)? If acting out of fear, ask yourself what is the worst thing that's likely to happen if you adopt a more positive approach. If you think you can handle the least desirable possibility, then consider switching from the fear-based course.

Spontaneous Change

Spontaneous remissions can occur with emotional problems as well as with physical ones. This happened to me about 15 years ago, when my almost lifelong fear of dogs simply vanished. Starting at about age three when a big dog jumped on me, I had a fear of dogs, especially large ones. I grew up in a rural area where many dogs were allowed to run loose. Sometimes I was threatened or chased by a dog, and once I was even bitten. Although it wasn't a serious injury, the experience was frightening. Whenever a large or rambunctious dog came near me, I would feel uncomfortable or downright afraid.

Years later when I was employed on a military base, in my office building I noticed a military policeman with a drug-detecting dog—a big, beautiful German shepherd. (It was common practice for the security force to periodically visit government buildings with drug-detecting dogs.) Rather than feeling wary of the creature, I was surprised to find I had a strong desire to pet it. I considered asking the policeman if I could pet his canine assistant, but my better judgment won out. (When working dogs are on the job, they aren't supposed to be treated like pets.) I was mystified by my uncharacteristic reaction, and later was even more surprised to discover it wasn't just a one-time thing. My fear of dogs had simply vanished!

About two years after this incident, I adopted a German shepherd puppy and developed a fondness for him that extended to most other dogs as well. Several years later, I "adopted" a wolf I visited every few months. Usually he would be with several other wolves (all were socialized to humans), and their preferred method of greeting people was to jump up and lick their faces. Here I was—a person who for most of her life had been afraid of large dogs that might jump on her—intentionally going into a situation in which *wolves* were jumping on her! Now I often stop people in the street and ask if I can pet their dogs. I still have a healthy fear of dogs that are acting threatening, but the inappropriate fear I experienced for so many years is completely gone.

I wish I could say precisely how I overcame my fear of dogs and give five easy steps for getting rid fears and phobias. Unfortunately, I don't know what caused this significant change. I didn't have any kind of therapy, nor did I have a positive experience with a dog that might have changed my attitude. Without my conscious awareness, something within me shifted markedly. The point of relating this story is to demonstrate that this type of change can occur easily—effortlessly, in fact.

Energy Psychology

Paying attention to what we are thinking enables us to become aware of thoughts that lead to stress and unhappiness, but we all have automatic reactions that bypass the mechanism of thought. A person with a phobia of thunderstorms, for example, may hear a loud thunderclap and immediately feel fear. Almost like pulling one's hand away from a hot surface, we react to certain stimuli without engaging our thought process. Energy psychology techniques are especially effective with these kinds of automatic reactions. They can eliminate (or at least diminish to manageable levels) emotional problems such as anxiety, fears, phobias, trauma, grief, guilt, anger, shame, addictive cravings, and even self-esteem issues. The methods also have been successful with physical problems including headaches, body pains, breathing difficulties, and allergies. With energy psychology, these seemingly intractable difficulties can be eliminated or reduced in severity—sometimes in as little as a few minutes—by following a few simple procedures. The techniques are noninvasive and inexpensive, and you can perform most of them yourself. Visiting a practitioner for short-term treatment is considerably less costly (and in many cases, faster and more effective) than most forms of psychological therapy. There are books and videos that provide detailed information on various energy psychology therapies; instructions for some methods are available for free on the Internet.

Energy psychology is based upon the premise that emotional problems (as well as some physical problems) are characterized by disruptions in the body's energy field, and that these problems can be treated with methods that affect the energy field. Proponents of energy psychology don't claim the techniques work for everyone, but many who have used them have had excellent—sometimes phenomenal—results. The procedures can be effective in a single session, but often multiple sessions are needed.

Most of the techniques can be performed by yourself or with the help of a friend, but there can be great value in consulting a skilled practitioner. The key to effectiveness is accurately identifying the issues to be treated, and these issues are not always obvious. Emotional problems can be like an onion, with many layers that need to be peeled away before you reach the core. A skilled practitioner can be invaluable in identifying these issues, as well as instructing you in the correct use of the procedures. It also should be noted that there are reasons we manifest physical and emotional problems; they don't just happen by chance. Eliminating the symptoms without identifying or addressing the cause(s) is likely to result in a return of the original problem or a manifestation of it in another form.

Critics of energy psychology claim there is no scientific basis for this type of therapy and that it works only because the patient believes it will work. In my view, all therapies (including conventional medical treatments) are based upon belief systems, and energy psychology techniques are no exception. The fact that a method is based upon beliefs doesn't mean it won't work, nor does the lack of an explanation for how something works invalidate its effectiveness. Numerous pharmaceutical drugs have been effective despite the fact that when they were first developed, scientists could not explain how or why they worked.

Some energy psychology methods involve the use of affirmations, which I generally don't recommend by themselves. Although affirmations sound good in theory (no pun intended), typically all you're doing is reminding yourself of—and reinforcing—what you truly believe, which usually is the opposite of the affirmation. When incorporated into energy psychology procedures, however, affirmations can be helpful.

Energy psychology is a rapidly evolving field; quite a few methods are available and more are being developed. Here I will briefly cover two techniques that have significantly helped many people. Please note that these are not necessarily the most effective methods for all individuals; they simply are the ones I'm most knowledgeable about. You may find that another modality works as well or better for you.

Thought Field Therapy

In the methods collectively known as Thought Field Therapy (a term coined by Roger J. Callahan, Ph.D., who first developed the technique), energy field disruptions can be corrected by tapping on acupressure points while the person being worked on "tunes in" to his or her problem. One of the most widely used forms of Thought Field Therapy is Emotional Freedom Techniques (EFT), which was developed by Gary Craig. The EFT website (*www.emofree.com*) has a wealth of information, including specific instructions for performing the techniques. The EFT mailing address is P.O. Box 1393, Gualala, California 95445 USA.

Not long after I learned about EFT, I was visiting a friend's family and had the opportunity to use the method with Sara, a 39-year-old woman who had been afraid of dogs since she was bitten by one as a child. Less than a year before our visit, her husband had adopted a friendly and energetic Labrador retriever. Sara felt very nervous around the dog, and at one point had given her spouse an ultimatum: "It's either me or the dog." Things improved after the Lab went through obedience training, but the situation was still tenuous. It was apparent that Sara's husband dearly loved his canine friend; it would have broken his heart to give him up. The night before I was leaving, I told Sara about EFT and offered to download and print the EFT manual from the Internet for her. Although she thought the whole thing was a bit odd, she was open-minded and motivated enough to try anything that might help. Sara's husband stood by as she and I went through the tapping sequences. From the look on his face, I was sure he must think I was a nutcase but was too polite to say so.

It was several months before I got any feedback on the effectiveness of the EFT treatment on Sara. In a phone conversation with my friend, Sara's husband mentioned that her fear of dogs seemed to have disappeared. The last I heard, the family had adopted a second dog (a miniature poodle) because Sara wanted a dog of her own!

PSYCH-K

The energy psychology therapy known as PSYCH-K was developed by psychotherapist Robert M. Williams, M.A. after several years of research and working with thousands of individuals and groups. The method is believed to increase communication between the two brain hemispheres and facilitate direct communication with the subconscious mind, enabling people to alter their beliefs and maximize their potential. PSYCH-K uses muscle testing and other techniques to identify beliefs and access the subconscious mind to achieve desired changes. It can be used to make changes in a broad range of areas, including self-esteem, relationships, health, body image, prosperity, personal power, and grief and loss. For more information on PSYCH-K, refer to the PSYCH-K website (*www.psych-k.com*) or contact the PSYCH-K Centre at P.O. Box 548, Crestone, Colorado 81131 USA.

I'm very much in favor of self-help techniques, but there are times when a skilled practitioner can be of great help. A few years ago, I had a PSYCH-K session with Rob Williams that turned out to be a good example of the value of consulting a professional. Starting with my stated problem, in about 20 minutes of conversation, he distilled it down to the core issue I really needed to address—which was completely different from the issue I had initially presented. Incorrectly identifying the underlying issue is one of the most common reasons for lack of results with the do-it-yourself approach to energy psychology. Unfortunately, when people try one of the methods on their own without much success, they are likely to give up on energy psychology entirely and miss out on this valuable resource. For those who are ready to make significant personal changes, energy psychology techniques can be effective tools.

Part III
Physical Strategies

6

Health Without Hype

"Preserving health by too severe a rule is a worrisome malady."
—Francois de La Rochefoucauld

Health Responsibility

To introduce this chapter, I'd like to make it clear that I am simply sharing my views, not telling readers how to live their lives. A fundamental concept of my philosophy is that each of us is totally responsible for our own well-being. If we choose to follow someone's advice (whether that person is a doctor, an author, or a stranger on the street), it's a choice *we* have made. This idea flies in the face of the victim mentality so pervasive in our over-litigated society. Yet until we can accept full responsibility for our bodies and our lives, we will continue to align with widely held beliefs that lead to poor health and age-related degeneration. It is crucial to recognize and pay attention to your own beliefs rather than denying them and pretending they don't exist. Some of the health-related ideas in this book may not be appropriate for some individuals because they conflict with their present beliefs. As in all other areas of your life, where health is concerned, follow your own inner guidance.

As mentioned in the Introduction, I intentionally chose not to provide scientific validation for all of the health-related information in this book. Quantum physics has proven that the observer affects that which is observed, so there is no such thing as a truly "objective" study. Prevailing beliefs about what is beneficial or detrimental to our health shift radically from year to year. Substances as diverse as soy products, coconut oil, eggs, potatoes, and coffee are demonized one year and exalted the next (or vice-versa). Where I present a product or practice as preferable to others, I note that the recommendation is based on a belief rather than an absolute truth. *All* such recommendations—regardless of the source—are based upon beliefs. The crucial factor is whether or not you align with those beliefs.

Health Care Services

As a general rule, I avoid doctor visits and diagnostic tests as much as possible. A few years ago, I started noticing that when I had a medical checkup and told the doctor I had no health concerns, he seemed a bit uneasy. It was apparent that he *wanted* to find something wrong. Almost instinctively, wanting to give the doctor what he was looking for, I would find myself trying to think of every little health issue I'd ever had. Focusing on past problems of any kind is not only unhelpful, it's counterproductive—it reinforces the problems and makes them more likely to recur. The doctor's intention was not to cause me harm in any way; in fact, he wanted to help me. According to his training and beliefs, there almost certainly had to be something wrong (or about to go wrong) with the health of a person over age 30. He simply wanted to find the problems and treat them to the best of his ability. Like virtually all medical doctors in our society, he was taught that disease and dysfunction is the norm and that a person in perfect health is an anomaly.

There have been times I've felt that going the conventional medical route was the right thing to do; at other times I felt it wasn't. For example, during a routine checkup in 1992, my doctor found what he thought were enlarged lymph nodes in my lower abdomen. Since I had no gynecological problems that might have affected nearby lymph nodes, he was almost certain this was an indication of non-Hodgkin's lymphoma (cancer of the lymphatic system) and wanted me to have a biopsy. The early symptoms of that disease are rather vague. I did have some of the symptoms (fatigue, chills, and itchy skin), but they could just as easily have been due to working in cold office in the wintertime in a job I disliked. I researched the disease and discovered that the recommended treatment was so harsh that it probably would have killed me before the cancer did. (I have severe reactions to virtually all medications that can cause nausea.) The biopsy would have damaged the lymph nodes even if they turned out to be healthy. If I wasn't going to take the treatment anyway, I figured there was no point in having a biopsy, so I refused it. Also, my gut feeling was that I did not have lymphoma.

To protect himself against a possible lawsuit, the doctor documented his preliminary diagnosis and recommendations and sent them to me in a letter. (Considering the number of lawsuits against medical professionals, I couldn't blame him.) The bottom line is that I never had the biopsy, and I'm still very much alive and healthy. When I had another checkup a couple of months later, the suspicious lumps were no longer there. If I had gone through with the biopsy, I would now have damaged lymph nodes.

Despite the statistics that supposedly prove the value of various diagnostic tests, I choose not to subject myself to cholesterol screenings, mammograms, and other disease detection measures considered mandatory for health-conscious adults. If you look hard and often enough for something, you're likely to create it eventually. It's normal for the human body to produce some irregular cells; the vast majority of the time, it destroys them on its own. I've long suspected that early detection methods for breast cancer are part of the reason the rates of this disease have skyrocketed. When a mammogram reveals a small cluster of "malignant" cells, doctors immediately take action with surgery, radiation, and/or chemotherapy. These assaults to the body weaken the immune system, which then allows the cancer to take hold. If doctors hadn't interfered, the body might well have destroyed the abnormal cells on its own. The "cancer victim" would have remained healthy and been spared great physical and emotional (as well as financial) trauma.

For a person with a fear of getting cancer and a strong belief in the conventional medical system, however, this approach may not be the best one. It is imperative that you feel good about the choices you are making. Not buying into the cancer industry in any manner makes me feel healthy and empowered, but if it would make you feel scared and vulnerable, then recognize and heed those feelings. If you believe you need to go for medical checkups, then by all means do so. Nonetheless, it might serve you well not to completely dismiss the ideas presented here, which may prove helpful to you at some point.

Holistic and Conventional Medicine

Conventional Western medicine is excellent for treating traumatic injuries, cardiac arrest, acute infections, and other medical crises. I feel fortunate to have access to medical professionals and services that can handle these problems so effectively. When addressing chronic, long-term health issues, however, conventional medicine often falls short. The use of drugs and surgery for treating conditions like cardiovascular problems and cancer frequently produces less than satisfactory results. The treatments themselves often cause additional health problems.

Holistic medicine emphasizes the importance of the whole and interdependence of its parts; the term is used to describe more natural alternatives to conventional medical therapies. Increasingly, the line of demarcation between the practice of conventional and holistic medicine is blurring. Chiropractors traditionally have had a holistic philosophy, but a growing number of conventionally trained medical doctors are becoming more holistic in their approach (and more willing to use alternative therapies). Conversely, some practitioners of alternative medicine are becoming *less* holistically oriented. This trend may be due to the requirements of managed care insurance systems, many of which now cover some alternative therapies.

My contrasting experiences with acupuncturists illustrates how differently various individuals can practice the same modality. More than 10 years ago, I had a series of acupuncture treatments from a doctor of Oriental medicine whose background included several years of training and experience in China. He didn't just focus on the problem I had consulted him for, but used a variety of diagnostic techniques (such as pulse and tongue analysis) to identify other imbalances. I found him to be highly skilled and very thorough.

Last year when I consulted another acupuncturist, my experience was markedly different. This practitioner was a doctor of Oriental medicine who served on the faculty of an acupuncture school and had several years of training and practice in China. I was seeking help for chronic neck and upper back pain, as well as some other energy imbalances I thought might be improved with acupuncture. During the first visit, I was astonished when the doctor quickly scanned the forms I'd filled out, asked me a few general questions, and immediately started treatment. Without so much as taking my pulse (an important diagnostic step that involves far more than the Western method of pulse-taking), he had me lie down on the table and inserted a few needles in my neck and back. As the doctor scurried from one treatment room to the next, it seemed that his primary concern was to shuttle as many patients through his office as quickly as possible. In my estimation, this doctor was not practicing holistic medicine; he was practicing conventional medicine with needles!

A few weeks later, I consulted a chiropractor for the same problems and was favorably impressed with his thorough diagnostic approach, detailed explanations, and comprehensive treatment program designed to achieve lasting improvements. The point I'm making here is not that one type of treatment is superior to another; both acupuncture and chiropractic care (as well as most other modalities) can be effective when applied correctly and appropriately. My intention is to show that the health care world is changing so fast that it's best not to make blanket judgments about the value of one method over another. My disappointing experience with the acupuncturist served to teach me that my preconceptions about various kinds of health treatments were no longer valid.

Particularly for treating chronic (rather than acute) health issues, my personal preference is for holistic treatments because they are considerably less invasive and more natural to the body. However, it should be noted that the use of nutritional supplements, herbs, and other holistic treatments follows the same paradigm as the use of drugs and surgery. With both conventional and holistic medicine, we are using something outside of ourselves to facilitate healing. Conventional medical treatments are not "bad" when used appropriately.

When I represented a nutritional products company, I often heard the management describe the pharmaceutical industry as if it were made up of villains who were out to take people's hard-earned money and make them dependent upon harmful drugs. Conversely, the nutritional supplement companies were depicted as health saviors operating solely from a desire to help people. Having previously been employed by a pharmaceutical company, I had a more balanced view. Pharmaceutical companies do promote the use of drugs way beyond what I think is beneficial, yet they too (in alignment with their own beliefs, which are very different from mine) have a fundamental intention of helping people. Certainly that was true of the individuals I interacted with in the nearly two years I worked at the company. And yes, pharmaceutical drugs often do more harm than good, but in some cases they're lifesaving. Regarding the profit-related motivations of various industries, all companies (other than charities and not-for-profit organizations) are in business to make money. There's nothing wrong with that.

What the management of the nutritional products company failed to recognize is that both they and the pharmaceutical companies are operating from the same fundamental belief: that we must take certain substances to maintain or regain our health. Ultimately I chose to disassociate myself from the nutritional company not because of the products, which were of high quality, but due to its marketing approach. I was drawn to the business initially because I liked both the products and the fact that nearly everyone I met at the company was motivated by the desire to help people improve their health and well-being. Then the company started promoting their anti-aging supplements by telling potential customers that no matter how good they might look and feel at the moment, if they are over the age of 30, their bodies are "crumbling from the inside out." In my view, the fear-based marketing messages would do more harm than the products did good. Unfortunately, fear-based marketing is widely used in numerous industries because it's often very successful.

There is nothing wrong with using conventional or holistic health services and products; they are useful tools. The crucial point is to realize they are *only* tools—something to help us believe we can heal ourselves, which we have the ability to do on our own.

Why Treatments Don't Work

Individuals' reactions to all types of treatments are tremendously influenced by their expectations. When we are ready to make a change, we will draw into our experience something that enables us to believe we can make that change. For instance, a person who is ready to be relieved of an allergy will find a treatment (it could be anything from acupuncture to allergy shots) that will seem to eradicate it, or at least successfully treat the symptoms. I use the term "seem to" because the person actually got rid of the allergy herself—and had the ability to do so with or without treatment.

Conversely, someone who is not ready to be relieved of a health problem will have disappointing (or at best, temporary) results from any sort of treatment. Why, you may wonder, would anyone *not* want to get rid of a health problem such as an allergy? There are many possible reasons. Perhaps the allergy gives the person a reason not to engage in certain activities, or it reinforces his view of himself as a sensitive person. The allergy may be an external representation of the inner sensitivity he feels toward his environment. In many cases, longstanding health and personal problems are incorporated by the ego as part of its identity. If you continue to think of yourself as a person with allergies, it's unlikely you'll get rid of them completely unless you change your self-image.

In both conventional and holistic medicine, there has been an increasing awareness that mental and emotional factors play a role in disease and healing. Regrettably, this realization has led to an artificial separation in which some health problems are considered physical (due to faulty genes, bad luck, or an unhealthy lifestyle) and others are believed to be—at least partially—mental or emotional in origin. People with problems in the latter category (as well as those deemed to have a poor lifestyle) often feel their illness is somehow their fault. In truth, all health problems—including infectious diseases and injuries—start first in the mind. Everything in our experience we create internally and project into the physical world—which includes our bodies. I prefer to eliminate the "fault and blame" question entirely because it's irrelevant and counterproductive. If each of us has created everything in our experience, then *all* of it is "our fault"! Passing judgment on ourselves and others serves no useful purpose.

An obvious question is why someone would choose experiences that are painful, traumatic, or unpleasant. If we have a choice, then why don't all of us create a life that's easy and enjoyable? One might as well ask why everyone who goes to college doesn't choose to major in an easy subject. Most of us have life intentions that are best served by having some challenging experiences. For instance, a woman I met named Shari has overcome numerous health problems—including a life-threatening disease—without resorting to radical medical treatments. Several years ago, Shari was diagnosed with a severe case of Graves' disease, a thyroid disorder. Her doctor said it was imperative that she have the malfunctioning gland removed right away, but Shari refused surgery and opted to try a variety of holistic treatments (including energy healing and nutritional therapy) instead. Her doctor called her a fool and told her, "Go home to die." Despite the physician's dire prognosis, less than a year later, Shari was free of the disease. She now spends much of her time helping others heal themselves physically and emotionally, significantly improving the quality of their lives. Presuming Shari came into this lifetime with an intention to assist people with healing, it makes sense that she would have chosen to experience a serious health problem herself.

If everything were easy and trouble-free, it's likely that most of us would get bored. Also, there's value in contrast: a warm, sunny day seems even better after a week of cold rain. I've never appreciated being alive and well more than right after the few times I've survived a life-threatening experience. Several years ago, after a serious car accident that I walked away from without injury, I refused offers for a ride home from work. Instead I chose to walk for 20 minutes to the nearest subway station simply because I *could*. Despite my sore muscles (from tensing up during the accident), I enjoyed every step of that walk.

Why Health Problems Occur

Injuries and illnesses don't just happen by chance or because a person was exposed to disease-causing organisms. A health problem can be viewed as a signal, a message from the inner self. In many cases, the nature of the communication can be determined simply by considering what the affected area of the body represents. Lower back discomfort frequently indicates a lack of support, while pain in the upper back and shoulders may reflect a person's feeling that life is a burden. Foot problems can reveal a fear of moving forward; knee problems may reflect a lack of flexibility in the personality. Some associations are humorous. Urinary tract infections, for instance, commonly are a sign that the sufferer is "pissed off" about something. (When I developed a urinary tract infection and a blocked tear duct in the same week, I could only conclude that I must be pissed off and holding back tears!) One man noticed that the back of his neck ached whenever he had to deal with a client he thought of as "a pain in the neck." A writer who couldn't possibly have been pregnant had symptoms of pregnancy that perplexed her—until she realized they were a representation of the book she was trying to "birth." A helpful resource for determining the meaning and potential causes of various health conditions is Louise L. Hay's classic little book, *Heal Your Body*[19] The descriptions aren't necessarily appropriate for every health condition (each of us has our own internal "language"), but the book is a good starting point.

Communications from the inner self also can manifest in our environment, particularly in homes and automobiles. Since water often represents emotions, plumbing problems frequently relate to emotional issues. (A clogged pipe may reflect an emotional block, for example.) When a friend of mine was looking for a home in a new area, he noticed that every house he looked at had mold in the crawl space, as did the house he had just sold (which shouldn't have been prone to mold because it was in an area with low humidity). My friend also suffered from yeast-related problems in his body. After rejecting yet another potential house due to mold problems, he realized the mold and yeast were indications of festering emotional issues he'd been holding onto since early childhood.

A good example of this type of correspondence is the time I developed a painful muscle knot in the back of my right shoulder that was paralleled by a squeaking sound from the right side of my car's front axle. (When you compare the human body to an automobile, the right shoulder corresponds to the right front wheel area.) I noticed that the squeak was loudest when the shoulder was most painful. When the pain was mild, the squeak was hardly noticeable. I took the car to the dealer to have it repaired. A mechanic replaced and oiled the bearings, but the squeak did not improve—nor did my shoulder. According to Louise Hay in *Heal Your Body*, "Shoulders represent our ability to carry our experiences in life joyously. We make life a burden by our attitude."[20] When I read the description, it made sense. I had been thinking of the responsibilities of life as a burden; everything seemed like a hassle. I set an intention to adjust my attitude, and my shoulder felt a little better. Then I took the car back to the dealer, where a top-notch mechanic was assigned to the job. It took him several hours to identify the problem and fix it. Rather than being annoyed that the repair was taking longer than expected, I felt sorry for the mechanic. Unbeknownst to him, he was dealing with more than just a simple squeak! This time when I got the car back, the annoying sound was gone. Within a few days, the pain in my shoulder went away as well. Getting the car repaired did not alleviate my shoulder problem, of course. What happened was that when I stopped looking at life as a burden, my attitude change was reflected in both my car and my shoulder.

We typically view illnesses and physical discomfort as negative, but this isn't necessarily the case. For most of my life, I've perceived muscle soreness from exercise or bodywork to be a positive sign—it means I'm getting stronger or becoming more flexible, or that constricted areas are returning to their normal state. The soreness may be uncomfortable, but it doesn't really bother me—in a way, it feels good. Illnesses, however, I perceived as negative—they were caused by foreign invaders that mercilessly attacked my body. If pathogens overcame my defenses and made me sick, I thought the best course of action was to try to fight them off. In fact, viruses and other pathogens are present in our bodies at all times; we just aren't aware of them until they proliferate and cause noticeable effects, which we label *illness*. What I failed to recognize is that these organisms serve a useful purpose, which is why our bodies allow them to be present. Symptoms such as mucous discharge, fever, sweating, and diarrhea are part of the body's cleansing process—the body's version of a major housecleaning. To halt these processes with medication is counterproductive to the maintenance of health and balance.

A couple of months after having this insight, I came down with the flu, which gave me the opportunity to observe how my new perspective affected my experience of illness. While I wasn't happy about the sore throat, congestion, fever, chills, and muscle aches, I chose to accept these symptoms as part of a necessary and beneficial process. Overall, the illness turned out to be considerably milder than all the other times I've had the flu. Of course, I don't know for sure that the severity of the illness was affected by the change in my attitude, but I suspect it was. To quote an adage, "Whatever we resist, persists."

Energy Healing

Energy healing can be broadly defined as "restoring to a state of balance (health) by means that affect the body's nonphysical energy centers and energy field." This description covers a wide variety of approaches that range from acupuncture to Therapeutic Touch (a form of laying-on-of hands) and numerous other practices.

In energy therapies such as laying-on-of-hands (that is, methods that do not involve the use of tools such as acupuncture needles or electronic devices), the "healer" generates a certain vibration and directs it to the "healee." If the healee allows it, his body entrains to that vibration, resonance occurs, and the healee's system returns to its natural state. To use a musical analogy, it's as if the healee is singing off-key and can't find the right pitch. The healer is singing on key, and sings the note strongly until the healee is able to match the note and maintain it on his own. In cases where the healer temporarily takes on some of the symptoms of the healee, it's as if the healer has wavered from the note and gone off-key along with the healee.

I used quotations marks around "healer" and "healee" (a term I coined as an alternative to *patient*) because no one can heal another person—we can only heal ourselves. Those we think of as healers (whether in conventional or holistic disciplines) are actually facilitators that assist other people in healing themselves. This fact should in no way minimize the importance of energy healers' work. Not only is energy healing just as "real" as conventional medical methods, it works on a more fundamental level. There are numerous cases in which an energy healer facilitated the cure of a condition medical professionals had given up on. If I were unable to manage a serious or chronic health problem on my own, my personal preference would be to try energy healing prior to seeking help from a conventional medical practitioner. All too often, people consult an energy healer as a last resort, after their bodies have suffered damage from invasive medical treatments.

As with any health care professional, use discernment when selecting an energy healer, both with the method and the practitioner. Personal recommendations can be valuable, but the most important factor is following your own intuition.

In addition to the plethora of energy healing services offered by trained practitioners, there are energy therapies that do not require the services of a professional. With simple instructions, most people can perform the techniques themselves. One popular and easy-to-use energy healing method is *acupressure*, the practice of applying pressure to specific points (commonly called acupuncture points) on the surface of the body to increase energy, alleviate pain, and restore the body to optimal functioning. Acupressure is sometimes called *reflexology*, although the latter term is more often used to refer specifically to acupressure performed on the feet and hands. A good resource for learning acupressure is the book *Body Reflexology: Healing at Your Fingertips* by Mildred Carter and Tammy Weber.[21]

A Healthy Environment

The information we read and hear regarding what is good and bad for our health is based upon beliefs, and in this book I've made a sincere effort to avoid presenting beliefs as absolute truths. However, many beliefs regarding health are so strongly held in collective consciousness that it's difficult not to align with them, at least to some degree. It also should be noted that "collective consciousness" is not something outside of ourselves that we are passively subject to. Each of us participates in and contributes to collective consciousness, which is why it is called "collective." When even one individual alters her beliefs, the change affects collective consciousness.

I sometimes refer to our strongly held mass beliefs as "the default." It's certainly possible for an individual to override the default, and many have done so. In *The Holographic Universe*, Michael Talbot presents numerous examples of documented cases of people who defied what are considered to be fundamental laws of nature. Yet most of us would find it hard to accomplish feats like surviving for years without food or water, as did German mystic Therese Neumann.[22] Nor could we handle poisonous snakes and drink strychnine (rat poison) and remain unharmed, which is a common practice for some members of Pentecostal Christian churches in the southeastern United States. We can, however, choose to be unaffected by whatever the media is focusing on as the latest scare this month.

A poignant example of how health fears can adversely affect a person's life is a woman I met who confided in me her terror of asbestos. On one occasion, for a short period of time, she was exposed to a low level of asbestos in an office where old ceiling tiles were being replaced. Although her exposure was so minimal that asbestos experts assured her there was no risk to her health, she was plagued by fears she knew were irrational. This healthy, vibrant woman was worrying herself sick over something harmless to her! She isn't alone. More and more, I've noticed people doing this sort of thing. They align with a well-publicized belief about the dangers of something and focus on it to the point that their fear—not the actual substance or disease, but their fear of it—adversely affects their daily life.

How do these situations get started? Typically, they begin when a substance or disease is deemed to be a serious risk to our health and well-being. The media and numerous individuals focus on the purported dangers. We are reminded of it practically every time we look at a newspaper or turn on the radio or television news, and it peppers our conversations. In short order, an industry grows up around it: products and services are developed and marketed; and lawyers, health professionals, and insurance companies get involved. A few examples of these industries are cancer detection and treatment, AIDS testing and treatment, asbestos removal, and radon mitigation. What many of us fail to realize is that we don't have to buy into these beliefs and fears.

Tobacco

Beliefs about the harmful effects of certain substances are very strong and deeply ingrained in most individuals and in collective consciousness, to the point that the simplest option is to limit or avoid using them. Regarding tobacco, Americans have been inundated since the 1960s with data indicating that smoking cigarettes leads to several life-threatening diseases. It would be difficult for someone in the United States to be unaffected by that belief and smoke heavily for years with no adverse effects. If you can accomplish this (with tobacco or anything else), then more power to you. As I've said before, *you* are the ultimate authority on your own health and well-being.

When a friend who had been smoking for a couple of years was considering quitting, I encouraged her by appealing to her vanity. "Forget about lung cancer and emphysema," I said (only half-facetiously); "smoking can cause wrinkles and stain your teeth." In fact, smokers generally do look older than their nonsmoking contemporaries.

If you live with someone who smokes and it bothers you, arrange to have the person's smoking restricted to limited areas. Beyond that measure, I suggest that when nonsmokers find themselves near a person who is smoking, they ignore it as much as possible. What we focus on, we automatically attract. If you pay a lot of attention to being annoyed by smokers, I can almost guarantee you will encounter inconsiderate smokers more and more often. Although I've never smoked anything in my life, I acknowledge that other people have the right to make their own choices.

Pharmaceutical and Over-the-Counter Drugs

Pharmaceutical drugs are best reserved for short-term use (in cases of acute infection, for example). For chronic health issues, investigate other methods of healing that will do more than treat the symptoms. If you've been given a prescription, particularly for a drug you expect to take long term, it's worthwhile to learn all you can about it. Read the literature that comes with your prescription and do further research (on the Internet or in recently published books or periodicals) to obtain information from sources other than the manufacturer.

Don't take antibiotics unless you have a bacterial infection or are undergoing surgery that may predispose you to infection. This suggestion may seem obvious, yet doctors frequently prescribe antibiotics to treat viral illnesses. Antibiotics not only kill the bacteria that cause infections, these drugs also destroy the beneficial bacteria in the intestines that are needed for proper digestion. After completing a course of antibiotics, it's a good idea to replace these essential bacteria (often called *probiotics*) by eating yogurt or taking a broad-spectrum probiotic supplement. For at least two weeks after finishing the antibiotics, have two or three servings per day of plain, unsweetened, organic yogurt (which contains probiotics). Soy-based yogurts are an option for those who don't use dairy products. People who don't like yogurt can opt for probiotic supplements, which are available in natural foods stores.

Most over-the-counter drugs only treat symptoms and can actually impede healing. For example, reducing a fever can slow your recovery because fever helps the body combat pathogens. Cold remedies that stop a runny nose can hinder the body's cleansing process and cause side effects such as drowsiness or nervousness. I prefer to keep no over-the-counter drugs in my home other than a pain reliever for occasional use.

A Healthy Home

Toxins commonly found in homes include impurities in the water supply, as well as toxic chemicals in household cleaners, pesticides, and herbicides. Here are some suggestions for minimizing toxins in your home:

- Drink filtered water (preferably from a reverse osmosis system) or water from a natural spring or well. Tap water from municipal sources usually contains chlorine, added fluoride, and other contaminants. It also doesn't taste very good.
- Install chlorine-removing water filters in all showers and bathtubs. Chlorine is absorbed through the skin, and showering in chlorinated water releases fumes that are absorbed through the lungs. Filtering the water you bathe in can noticeably improve the condition of your hair and skin.

- Replace toxic cleaning products with natural alternatives such as natural liquid soap (for basic cleaning), vinegar (for cleaning and disinfecting), baking soda (for cleaning and deodorizing), salt (for cleaning and polishing), and hydrogen peroxide (for disinfecting).
- Avoid using herbicides, and minimize the use of pesticides as much as possible. If you must use a pesticide, opt for the least toxic alternative.

It's worthwhile to minimize exposure to toxins in your daily environment (including your workplace, if possible), but don't get too upset about occasional exposures. The stress from worrying about them may do more damage to a healthy person than the toxin itself. As with anything else, notice and heed your body's communications. Move away from things that bother you, which can include not just toxic substances, but people and situations you find stressful. As a general rule, however, consider yourself invulnerable to these influences—and you will be.

7

Nutrition Without a Diet Plan

○ ○

"Always take a good look at what you're about to eat. It's not so important to know what it is, but it's critical to know what it was."

—*Unknown*

What (and When) to Eat

Dietary recommendations typically are based on the assumption that most people's nutritional requirements are pretty much the same, which clearly is not the case. Everyone with a digestive system is an alchemist—we transmute the foods we eat into completely different substances, which can vary tremendously from person to person. The adage "One man's meat is another man's poison" (attributed to the Roman philosopher Lucretius) is sometimes literally true.

For many years, I've done a great deal of research and read numerous books on nutrition and diet. Ultimately I came to the conclusion that nobody has "the answer" to the question of optimum diet, simply because there isn't one. A couple of years ago I read three books on a well-established health and nutrition system; each of the books was authored by a recognized expert in the field. I was amused to find significant contradictions in the information given by the three experts, and this was within the same system! Various systems can be helpful as a starting point, but ultimately it is the individual who is the true expert. For this reason, most of the suggestions about nutrition in this book are general in nature. My intention is not to create yet another belief system about diet.

The optimum diet for each individual is matching food choices to the individual's vibrational quality. The best way to do this is to pay attention to your preferences and how particular types of food affect you. Notice the way you feel after eating various foods and how they affect your digestive system. We change constantly, so it's important to be open to trying new foods and varying your diet. Foods that were your favorites a few years ago might not be appropriate for you now.

To make optimal food choices, get in tune with your body by paying attention to what (and when) you truly feel like eating. Unfortunately, sometimes it's hard to tell the difference between an intuitive feeling that you need a particular food and a craving based on an unhealthy dependency. (It's possible to become dependent on a substance like refined sugar, which affects some people like a drug.) A good method is to ask yourself not only what you feel like eating, but also how you *expect to feel* after you have eaten a food. If you don't think you will feel good after eating it, then don't eat it. Consume only foods you feel positive about putting into your body. Do you really want that processed snack—laden with synthetic flavor, artificial color, and preservatives—to become part of you?

All that being said, it's of the utmost importance to enjoy what you eat, so don't choke down something objectionable just because it's supposed to be good for you. Personally, I like eating desserts (including chocolate), but prefer a moderate amount of a high-quality treat rather than a large amount of something I consider junk food. Enjoying a few premium cookies or a slice of homemade cherry pie is far different from furtively bolting down a bag of greasy potato chips or synthetic-tasting candy.

Regarding diet and aging, the theory with the most supporting evidence is that eating a smaller quantity of food leads to decreased degeneration and greater longevity. This doesn't mean you should starve yourself, but erring on the side of smaller portions is a good idea. Eat when you are hungry and only when you are hungry, regardless of what time it is. Following set mealtimes is simply a convention. It takes about 20 minutes for the body to produce signals of fullness, so stop eating before you feel full. Eat several small meals throughout the day rather than one or two large ones. When you consume a large quantity of food at one sitting, more of it is stored as fat than if you had eaten the same amount at different times throughout the day.

Stuffing yourself with food is not a good practice, but neither is habitually ignoring hunger signals and repeatedly going for long periods without eating. (However, an occasional one-day fast can be beneficial for people without serious health problems.) Skipping meals in an effort to lose weight is counterproductive. When you don't have nourishment for several hours and are feeling strong hunger pangs, chemical messages alert your brain that you are in danger of starving. The next time you eat, your body will try to conserve as many calories as possible as a hedge against starvation.

The digestive process begins in the mouth. Take small bites, chew slowly, and pay attention to the flavor and texture of what you are eating. Avoid watching television or engaging in intense conversations while you are eating. (Postpone heated debates until well after the meal.) Awareness of the eating process will enable you to feel satisfied with a smaller amount of food than if you bolted down your meal half-consciously.

Make an effort to get in a relaxed state before, during, and after eating. Avoid eating when you are feeling very stressed or upset. In stressful situations, the body shunts the blood supply away from the digestive organs, so a meal eaten when you are stressed will not be properly digested. If you pay attention, you probably will notice that eating when you are emotionally upset usually gives you indigestion.

Special Dietary Concerns

Vegetarianism Versus Nonvegetarianism

The human digestive system appears to have been designed for a primarily plant-based diet; our organs are more like those of an herbivore (an animal that feeds primarily on plants) than a carnivore (meat-eater). The digestive tract of carnivorous animals is short (about three times the length of the body) and relatively smooth, which facilitates rapid digestion. Human intestines are approximately 12 times the length of the body and are designed for slower digestion, which is necessary to break down and assimilate nutrients from plant matter. Our dental structure also is best suited to a plant-based diet. Most of our teeth are incisors (for cutting) and molars (for grinding) rather than the sharp canine teeth carnivores use to tear flesh. We do, however, have the capacity to digest and assimilate animal-based foods as well, and people in some cultures thrive on a diet that consists primarily of animal products. Vibrationally, the primary difference between foods derived from plants and those from animal sources is their density: animal-derived foods are denser than plants. I suspect that as humans continue to evolve, we will choose to consume more plant-based foods because we will become less compatible with the denser animal foods.

All forms of life, including plants, are sentient beings. In my view, it is not inherently wrong to consume animal-derived foods as long as the creatures that have given their lives for our nourishment are treated with respect, compassion, and appreciation. People of more "primitive" cultures hunted animals for food and their hides, but they did so with respect and appreciation for the creatures that gave their lives for the humans' nourishment, warmth, and shelter. Confining chickens to cages, veal calves to tiny pens, and cows to feed lots does not constitute "respect and compassion"!

If you choose to consume animal-derived foods, know the source of those foods. Factory-farmed beef, for instance, not only may contain hormones, antibiotics, and other contaminants, it has the vibrations of fear and suffering the animal endured during its life. Aside from the ethical implications of contributing to cruelty to animals by supporting such industries, do you really want this tainted meat to become part of your own body? Become—quite literally—a *conscious consumer.*

Genetically Engineered Foods

The concept of balance and harmony as a basic requirement is a belief that is fundamental to humankind. Technological alterations to nature are not inherently beneficial or harmful; it depends upon how well they fit into the larger scheme of things. In some cases, the indications are compelling that the eventual outcome is likely to be detrimental. Genetically engineered foods fall into this category. In foods with Genetically Modified Organisms (GMOs), a segment of the genetic code has been modified to enhance specific traits such as growth rate, appearance, flavor, shelf life, or resistance to disease or pests.

With genetic engineering of foods, an important factor to consider is that GMOs result in a loss of diversity within species—and diversity is fundamental to the way nature works. It's virtually impossible to prevent genetically altered plants from pollinating other plants; already there have been several cases in which organic crops were found to be contaminated by GMOs from genetically altered plants in nearby fields. Unexpected effects of GMOs have already become evident. (One of the most publicized cases is the death of monarch butterflies from genetically modified corn.) In addition, it's very likely that genetic modifications alter the vibrational quality—and therefore the nutritional value—of the plants in ways scientists do not yet understand.

The issue of GMOs in the food supply concerns me, yet I realize that giving attention to worst-case scenarios is counterproductive—it makes the dire possibilities more, not less, likely to occur. Rather than focusing on potential disasters, I find it more constructive to put my energy (and shopping dollars) into supporting companies not involved in any way with genetically altered foods.

Organic Foods

Other than growing all your own food (which is impractical for most of us), the best way to be sure you aren't getting foods with GMOs or pesticides is to buy products that are certified organic. At least at this point, your chances of avoiding GMOs are exponentially better if you choose organic foods. (As of this writing, most organic crops have not been contaminated with GMOs, and laws in the United States still uphold organic standards.) In addition, you won't be supporting the companies that are proponents of genetically engineered foods. Buy meat, eggs, dairy, and other animal products only from producers that treat the animals with respect. Such companies usually mention these policies on their product packaging.

Organically grown vegetables and fruits are actually more nutritious than those grown with pesticides. Plants use flavonoids (potent antioxidants with numerous health benefits) to protect themselves from insects. If pesticides are used, the plants are less likely to produce the highest levels of these nutrients. Comparison tests between organic and conventional fruits and vegetables consistently show flavonoid levels to be significantly higher in organic produce.

Organic and animal-friendly products often cost more than conventional ones, but the effects of supporting these companies extend far beyond your own dinner table. If you are inclined to settle for conventional rather than organic food due to the higher cost of organics, think of the extra dollars spent as a contribution to several worthy causes. Buying organics supports small, independent farms (the major suppliers of organic products), the well-being of farm workers (who won't be exposed to pesticides, herbicides, and chemical fertilizers), and the humane treatment of animals. Organic production systems preserve and restore natural ecosystems, keeping the soil, water, and air free from toxic chemicals. When you purchase from companies that operate with respect for humans, animals, and the environment, you are "voting with your wallet" to support these policies. As far as I'm concerned, this is by far the most effective type of voting.

Nutritional Sources

Plant Foods

Fresh fruits and vegetables contain a wide variety of vitamins, minerals, and other biologically active compounds such as flavonoids and carotenoids (plant pigments ranging from yellow to orange to red), many of which have yet to be isolated in laboratories. Like the flavonoids, carotenoids are potent antioxidants with numerous health benefits. Specific carotenoids such as lutein and zeaxanthin (both are found in high concentrations in kale, spinach, and other dark green leafy vegetables) are especially good for acute vision and eye health. Lycopene (found in red vegetables and fruits) is beneficial for the vascular system and has anticancer effects, particularly for prostate cancer. Anthocyanins (flavonoids in plant pigments ranging from blue to violet to red) have numerous benefits as well. The anthocyanins in blueberries can enhance brain function and help prevent cognitive decline. Ellagic acid (a phenolic compound found in fruits and nuts, particularly red raspberries) has antibacterial, antiviral, and anticancer properties; it also helps alleviate symptoms of gout. The chlorophyll in green plants has a chemical structure nearly identical to the hemoglobin in blood. In the body, chlorophyll acts an anti-inflammatory agent, promotes healthy bowel function, helps prevent infections, and neutralizes some carcinogens. If your daily diet doesn't include at least six servings of fruits and vegetables, consider using a whole food supplement made from high-nutrient plants.

Other plant foods that are beneficial to include in your regular diet are whole grains, beans, nuts, seeds, and sprouted seeds. Ground flaxseeds and flaxseed meal are excellent fiber sources that are high in omega-3 oils and easier to digest than bran or psyllium. (You can buy ground flaxseeds in natural foods stores, or purchase whole flaxseeds and grind them yourself.) There are many delicious whole grains besides the familiar wheat, rye, and barley. These lesser-known grains include quinoa (pronounced "keen-wa"), millet, kashi (buckwheat), spelt, and amaranth. For commercially prepared breads, an excellent option is a flourless, sprouted whole grain bread such as Ezekiel 4:9 Sprouted Grain Bread (available in the refrigerated section of natural foods stores).

Plant foods are best eaten raw or lightly cooked, as heat can change the vibrational quality of the food and destroy some of the nutrients. With some vegetables (such as broccoli and carrots), light cooking methods such as steaming can increase the bioavailability of nutrients by breaking down some of the cellulose in the cells walls. People unaccustomed to eating raw or lightly cooked foods should increase the proportion of these foods in their diet gradually to allow their digestive system to adjust to the change.

Essential Fatty Acids

Essential Fatty Acids (EFAs)—also known as omega-3, omega-6, and omega-9 oils—are necessary nutrients for the brain, eyes, skin, and hair, as well as for proper hormonal function. Low levels of EFAs can lead to a variety of health problems including dry skin, constipation, and depression. If you don't eat flaxseeds, hempseeds, oily fish (such as salmon), or other EFA-rich foods frequently, you can take EFA supplements in liquid or capsule form. If using fish oil, make sure the product label says it has been purified by molecular distillation, which is the most effective way to remove the impurities and toxins concentrated in fish oil.

Hempseed oil is the best plant-based source of a balanced array of all three types of omega oils. Unlike some fish oils, it also is environmentally friendly. Hempseed oil and hempseeds (a tasty and nutritious snack) have none of the mind-altering, drug-like effects of marijuana. In addition, hemp fiber is an ecologically excellent alternative to paper and cotton. Hempseed oil may be hard to find in stores, but it can be purchased by mail order. (To find a supplier, check with a natural foods store or perform an Internet search on "hempseed oil.") The Nutiva company offers organic food products including hempseed oil, shelled hempseeds, and hempseed food bars. Nutiva can be contacted by mail at P.O. Box 1716, Sebastopol, California 95473 USA; by phone at 707-823-2800 or 1-800-993-4367 (toll-free); or online at *www.nutiva.com*.

Sweeteners

A diet high in refined sugar can contribute to a variety of problems such as blood sugar disorders and mood swings. Refined sugar is listed in many different ways on product labels; some of the most common ones are corn syrup, brown rice syrup, fructose, and maltodextrose.

The artificial sweetener aspartame (brand name NutraSweet) tends to trigger a craving for sweet foods, which makes it ineffective as a weight loss aid and inappropriate for diabetics. Reactions to this substance vary greatly among individuals. Some people tolerate it without obvious ill effects, but in others it acts like a poison. With my first taste of aspartame, I knew it didn't agree with me and made a point of avoiding it. One time I inadvertently ate a cup of aspartame-sweetened yogurt. About an hour later, I had a sudden attack of headache, nausea, weakness, and dizziness so severe that I almost fainted in the floor. Most people don't react this strongly to the substance, but adverse reactions are not uncommon.

An excellent alternative to sugar and artificial sweeteners is stevia, which comes from the leaves of the stevia rebaudiana plant. Not only is stevia safe for diabetics, it contains compounds that can help regulate blood sugar. Stevia (which is available from natural foods stores in powder and liquid forms) also has antibacterial properties and can be used topically on the skin and gums. Honey is another good alternative to refined sugar. It has a high glycemic index (causes a rapid rise in blood sugar) and therefore is not appropriate for diabetics, but this effect is moderated when it is combined with other foods. Honey also has antibacterial properties and can be used topically to help heal wounds.

Nutritional Supplements

Nutritional supplements can be beneficial, but conventional vitamin and mineral pills are of questionable value. In many cases these products are not properly assimilated by the body, nor do they contain the cofactors and synergistic compounds found in whole foods. Researchers are continually discovering substances in foods that are beneficial to human health. These compounds work synergistically, so taking only those that have been identified and isolated into supplements does not provide complete nutrition. In addition, there is a vibrational, energetic quality to certain substances that nourishes our bodies, which is why synthetic supplements often don't do much good. They may simulate the chemical structure of selected nutrients, but they don't have the vibrational qualities of whole foods. Laboratory studies can demonstrate some of the biochemical effects, but we don't yet have instruments to measure the vibrational effects.

Superior alternatives to vitamin pills are whole food supplements made from high-nutrient foods such as wheat grass, barley grass, alfalfa, spirulina, chlorella, blue-green algae, deep-colored vegetables, dark-colored berries, and other nutrient-rich plants. High-quality brands of these products contain complete nutritional complexes the body can assimilate, as well as enzymes needed by the digestive system. There is a tremendous difference in the quality and ingredients of various brands of whole food supplements, so check labels carefully. Avoid products with added sweeteners (such as maltodextrose, barley malt, or brown rice syrup) or a significant amount of "filler" ingredients like flax meal, oat bran, rice bran, apple fiber, or lecithin.

Herbalism

There are countless varieties of herbs that are beneficial for various conditions or can be taken as tonics to promote overall wellness. Herbs certainly can be helpful, and I've used quite a few different kinds at various times in my life. They are, however, not a requirement for maintaining good health or youthfulness. Believing you must take herbs is just a couple of steps removed from believing you need pharmaceutical drugs to stay healthy.

Following are several herbs considered especially good for maintaining youthful well-being. The brief descriptions I've included are only a partial list of each plant's potential benefits. These herbs are available in natural foods stores and from mail-order nutritional products companies. Like most medicinal herbs, they are best taken at least half an hour before eating or two hours after a meal. Some of them also are available in herbal teas, which can be used at any time.

Ashwagandha (Winter Cherry)—In Ayurvedic medicine, ashwagandha is a tonic herb used to promote rejuvenation and longevity. It is known for a broad range of health benefits including reduced inflammation, enhanced brain function, improved stress management ability, and greater energy and vitality.

Bhringaraj (Eclipta Alba)—In Ayurvedic and Chinese medicine, bhringaraj is known for maintaining and enhancing hair color and fullness, improving skin, and rejuvenating teeth, bones, and vision.

Gotu Kola—In Ayurvedic and Chinese medicine, gotu kola (which does not contain caffeine) is known for improving circulation, strengthening collagen and connective tissue, enhancing hair strength and fullness, and promoting rejuvenation and longevity.

Gynostemma—A tonic herb widely used in Asia for promoting rejuvenation and longevity, gynostemma is known for a broad range of health benefits including greater energy and vitality, improved stress management ability, a stronger immune system, enhanced fat metabolism, and better digestion.

He Shou Wu (Fo Ti)—In Chinese medicine, he shou wu (which translates to "Mr. Wu's hair stays black") is known for maintaining and enhancing hair color and fullness, improving skin, and rejuvenating teeth, bones, and vision.

Horsetail (Shavegrass)—So named because the plant resembles a horse's tail, horsetail is known for promoting healthy skin, hair, nails, connective tissue, bones, and teeth. The herb contains high levels of the mineral silica, increases calcium absorption, and has diuretic properties.

Triphala—An Ayurvedic tonic for the digestive system, triphala (a blend of the fruits amalaki, bibhilaki, and haritaki) is known for normalizing bowel function and helping to detoxify and regenerate numerous body systems One of triphala's components, amalaki, is a natural source of vitamin C. Since triphala is an intestinal cleanser, start with a low dose (500 milligrams once or twice a day) and gradually increase the dose and/or frequency. If using triphala long term, take at least a one-week break from the supplement every month.

Wonderful Water

The importance to health of drinking an ample quantity of pure water can hardly be overemphasized. As a general rule, most people should drink two to three liters or quarts of purified water daily. For a rough estimate of the minimum number of ounces of water to drink daily, divide your body weight in pounds by two. (Example: 150 divided by 2 equals 75, so a person who weighs 150 pounds should drink at least 75 ounces of water per day.) Using the metric system, estimate one liter of water for every 30 kilograms of body weight. (Example: 75 kilograms divided by 30 kilograms equals 2.5, so a person who weighs 75 kilograms should drink at least 2.5 liters of water per day.) These formulas are not exact (the metric formula results in a slightly higher figure), but they give a general idea. Hot weather, strenuous exercise, and eating salty food increases your fluid requirements, sometimes markedly. People in high-altitude areas also need to drink more water.

Keep in mind that these quantity suggestions are general in nature and don't necessarily apply to everyone. The water present in foods counts too, and if you eat a lot of fruit or other water-heavy foods, you may not need to drink that much water. Like every other physical requirement, the need for water varies not just among individuals; it fluctuates in the same individual from day to day. Develop a sensitivity to your body's needs by noticing when you are thirsty, hungry, or sleepy. If you have become accustomed to not getting enough fluid and are in a continual state of dehydration, then thirst may not be an accurate indictor of how much water you need to drink. Unless you are already drinking a lot of water, try increasing your consumption (especially first thing in the morning) by one cup per day and notice if you feel better and have more energy.

I've discovered that when I feel fatigued for no apparent reason, it's often due to dehydration.

The body must warm up cold liquids before they can be absorbed, so it's best to drink water that is tepid or even warm. Cold drinks also can interfere with digestion, especially when taken with meals. Restaurants in the United States usually serve ice water, so make point of requesting water without ice when you're dining out. It can be beneficial to drink hot water occasionally because it has a cleansing effect on the system. To help alleviate constipation, drink a cup of hot water with lemon juice when you wake up in the morning. Do not, however, drink or cook with hot tap water, which contains dissolved impurities from the pipes and water heater.

It's best to drink water that comes from a natural well or has been distilled or filtered by reverse osmosis. Drink municipally supplied, unfiltered tap water only if filtered water is unavailable. Not only does most tap water contain chlorine, added fluoride, and other impurities, its unpleasant taste makes it less likely that you will drink an ample quantity.

Weight Management

Judging from recent news reports from numerous sources, the population in many industrialized countries keeps getting fatter. I suspect part of the reason for the increase in obesity is that many people are not getting adequate nutrition from their diets. In an effort to obtain needed nutrients, their brains keep sending messages that prompt them to eat more. Yet even people who eat a seemingly balanced diet of nutritious foods in reasonable quantities may tend to be overweight if these foods don't contain enough life force energy. Processed foods, factory-farmed meat, and fruits and vegetables picked too early are lacking in life force energy and do not truly provide nourishment. The overweight person's body thinks it is starving and adjusts to compensate, storing more calories as fat. This phenomenon may hold true even if the person consumes a moderate quantity of food and doesn't overeat. Conversely, when the body is given fresh food that was raised naturally and contains life force energy, the body knows it has been truly fed, and therefore maintains an appropriate weight.

Some people store too much fat for much the same reasons that others hoard money: the fear of future scarcity and the need for security. Those hoarding money may live a lifestyle of near-poverty, wearing old clothes, eating only inexpensive food, and avoiding spending for entertainment or vacations. They choose to live this way rather than dipping into their savings. Likewise, an overweight person may be chronically fatigued, yet unable to access the wealth of energy stored in his fat cells. In both cases, the underlying cause is a feeling of lack and fear of the future. However, if the money hoarder starts earning a good income and feels secure that it will continue, he might be more willing to loosen up and use some of his riches. In a similar fashion, if the overweight person starts giving his body the nutrients it needs, then his body may start using the accumulated fat stores.

As with age-related degeneration, body weight is inextricably linked to beliefs. If you believe you are basically an overweight person (or if the excess weight is serving a purpose for you), then you will not be thin. You may lose weight temporarily, but eventually you'll gain it back. Rather than following the latest diet fad, pay attention to your feelings, thoughts, and actions, which reveal your underlying beliefs. Remember that you have a choice of whether to continue to align with these beliefs.

8

Fitness Without a Regimen

○ ○

"People don't stop moving when they get old. People get old when they stop moving."

—*Unknown*

Don't Act Your Age

Being physically active is one of the most important things you can do to maintain or regain youthful functioning. It isn't necessary to join a health club, hire a personal trainer, or purchase expensive exercise equipment. Just move your body, and do it frequently.

Have you ever observed how children move when they're playing? They sit on the floor or the ground, jump up, run around, and flip over—an almost endless variety of actions and positions. Compare the movements of children and teenagers to those of adults. You'll observe that most adults move more slowly and stiffly, with a limited range of motion. When adults sit on the floor, many find it awkward and uncomfortable. Contrary to common belief, they lost their flexibility due to lack of use, not due to advancing age.

If you want to look and feel like a young person, then move like a young person. Replace some of the chairs in your home with large cushions, and sit on the floor regularly. Stay active all day long, not just during scheduled exercise periods. If you have a desk job, get up frequently and walk around. Visit coworkers personally rather than using the telephone or electronic mail. If you are restricted from leaving your work area, you still can get up from your chair and move around. People with jobs that require standing for long periods should look for opportunities to sit, even if it's on a countertop.

Develop an Exercise Habit

For those accustomed to a sedentary lifestyle, the habit of moving the body frequently may not come naturally at first. If you wait until you feel like exercising, you may not do it very often. Exercise is an area in which a regular routine serves most of us very well. Usually you'll find that once you take the first step, you will get into the mood of doing the exercise. Following are some suggestions for making exercise a regular part of your life:

- Establish a simple routine that includes some form of endurance (cardiovascular) exercise, stretching, and strengthening. It's best to start off with activities that don't require spending a lot of money on equipment or special clothing. With a minimal financial investment, you will feel free to move on to something else if the first activity you try doesn't suit you.

- Schedule a regular time for exercise. As a general rule, the earlier in the day you exercise, the better. Many people find it easier to adhere to a morning or noontime routine than one in the late afternoon or evening. As the day progress, the chances increase that something will interfere with your schedule.

- Use whatever means are necessary to motivate yourself: a workout buddy, exercise class, or fitness book or video. Most importantly, choose activities you enjoy. After getting past the initial discomfort of exercising when you aren't used to it, if you discover you genuinely don't care for a particular activity, then switch to another one—but don't quit exercising. Also, don't force yourself to exercise to the point that it becomes truly unpleasant or painful. Pushing too hard (especially at first) not only can lead to injuries, it can make you dread your next exercise session.

- Follow your new routine for three weeks, doing your best not to skip a scheduled session. It takes about 21 days to form (or break) a habit. By the end of the third week, you will be feeling—and perhaps seeing—the benefits of your fitness routine, and will want to continue it.

Some of the best exercises require the least paraphernalia. Brisk walking and jogging are endurance exercises that require only a good pair of shoes and supportive undergarments. For strengthening, you don't necessarily need to use weights or weight machines. The classic military-style pushup is an excellent strengthening exercise that involves no equipment. *Hatha yoga* (the branch of yoga that involves the practice of physical postures) is a comprehensive exercise system that stretches and strengthens muscles and connective tissue, improves balance and posture, and benefits internal organs. Despite the heavy marketing of yoga-related products, the practice requires only nonrestrictive clothing and a carpet or mat.

In addition to doing stretching exercises and maintaining flexibility, one of the best ways to prevent injuries is to avoid performing the same strenuous or high-impact activities on consecutive days. Skipping a day allows the body time for restoration and repair of any damage to muscles and connective tissue. It's a prevalent belief that people are more prone to injuries as they get older, but this isn't necessarily the case. In my teens and twenties, I rarely did any stretching and usually performed the same high-impact activities on consecutive days, which led to frequent minor injuries. Then I discovered I could maintain the same level of fitness by skipping days between workouts. I revised my fitness program to include stretching exercises and rest days, and also started performing different activities on alternate days. Consequently, I'm considerably less injury-prone now than when I was younger.

When your fitness habit is well established, periodically varying your routine can help keep it interesting. While it's beneficial and efficient to have habits that serve our purposes, there's a delicate balance between regularly following routines and being overly rigid. Exercising when you wake up in the morning is a great way to start the day, but occasionally you may want to give yourself a treat by just rolling out of bed and having a leisurely cup of tea.

Use Your "Other" Hand

Most of us tend to use our dominant hand (for about 90 percent of the population, it's the right hand) for tasks requiring fine coordination. Develop the habit of sometimes using your nondominant hand for eating, drinking, using a computer touch pad or mouse, throwing a ball, and other activities for which you normally would use your dominant hand. The right hand is connected to the brain's left hemisphere, which prefers structured information, letters, and symbols, is good at learning details and unrelated facts, and likes orderliness and predictability. The right hemisphere prefers pictures to letters or symbols, tends to learn the whole before the parts, and likes spontaneity and surprises. Ideally there should be a balance in our use of the two hemispheres, but modern culture and education tend to favor left-brain dominant activities. By using our nondominant hand, we can help activate the right hemisphere and balance our use of the various brain functions. (Note: In some left-handed people, the functions of the brain hemispheres are reversed from what is described above. It varies among individuals.)

The Tibetan Rites of Rejuvenation

Practices such as hatha yoga and *qi gong* (an ancient Chinese discipline that stimulates the flow of life force energy by using controlled breathing and movements) affect the subtle energies and benefit the mind and body. People who perform these practices regularly seem to age more slowly than their contemporaries. Although the techniques can be learned from books and videos, working with an instructor for initial training can be invaluable.

A practice I have found especially beneficial is the Tibetan Rites of Rejuvenation, a yoga-like routine brought to the West in the early 1900s by a British army colonel who spent several years in a Himalayan monastery. The practice became well known in the United States from a book called *Ancient Secret of the Fountain of Youth* by Peter Kelder.[23] The rites (often called the Five Tibetans, despite the existence of an optional sixth rite) are practiced around the world. They are believed to prevent aging by activating the body's nonphysical energy centers. The energy centers (also known as *chakras*) are associated with the endocrine glands. Impaired endocrine function is a significant factor in age-related degeneration, so keeping these glands working well helps maintain youthfulness.

There are numerous dramatic reports of rejuvenation and health improvements that have resulted from practicing the Five Tibetans. Kelder's book includes many impressive testimonials from people who report that after consistently practicing the rites for months or years, they look and feel as much as 20 years younger than they did before. These accounts may well have validity, but since I cannot personally attest to their accuracy, I have not included them here. Personally, I've found that practicing the Five Tibetans has increased my strength, flexibility, and balance. A month or so after I started the practice, I noticed that my senses of hearing and smell (which already were quite keen) became even sharper.

In addition to improving physical fitness and enhancing glandular functioning, practicing the Five Tibetans also has the advantage being fast (under 15 minutes per day), convenient (the routine can be performed almost anywhere and requires no equipment other than a carpet or mat), and cost-free (other than the possible purchase of a book).

Instructions for the Tibetan Rites

The rites consist of five different movements (with the addition of an optional sixth rite), each of which is performed 21 times. Start with three repetitions of each rite, adding two or three repetitions per week until you work up to the full 21. (As much as possible, do the same number of repetitions of all the rites.) The entire routine can be completed in less than 15 minutes. It is recommended that you perform the rites daily, missing no more than one day per week. Because the exercises are not high impact or overly strenuous, performing them daily does not lead to injuries.

The daily routine works well for many people, but for those who aren't likely to follow a daily schedule, it's better to practice the rites every second day than not at all. Another option is to do the full 21 repetitions on alternate days and perform only 7 repetitions on the days in between. Doing the routine sporadically, however, will not be effective. If you habitually miss two or more consecutive days, the benefits will diminish noticeably. If you are performing the rites daily, I recommend taking off at least one day a month. For women, the heaviest day of menstruation is a good day to skip.

In addition to following the instructions provided in this chapter, it's a good idea to read one of the books about the rites, which give complete directions and illustrations. *The Five Tibetans* by Christopher S. Kilham not only demonstrates and explains the rites; it provides instructions (which I've included below) for breathing during and between each rite.[24]

In Peter Kelder's book, the description of Rite 6 includes the practice of celibacy. This rite is presented as an optional addition to the other five rites; the exercise portion of Rite 6 is supposed to help control sexual desire.[25] Christopher Kilham says he doesn't believe celibacy is necessary for maintaining youthfulness, and I agree with him.[26] My view is that celibacy (while it is a choice of experience as valid as any other) is not a requirement for either rejuvenation or spiritual growth. I've found the exercise portion of Rite 6 to be helpful in strengthening abdominal muscles and organs, but it hasn't affected my libido at all (possibly because that isn't my intention for performing the rite).

Following is a concise version of the instructions for the Tibetan Rites of Rejuvenation. As with any other physical exercises, use common sense when performing the Five Tibetans. If you experience pain or dizziness, slow down or stop. Those under the care of a health professional for a serious condition (such as a heart problem) should check with that person prior to starting any exercise program, including this one.

Breathing—Prior to performing Rite 1 and after completing each rite, stand erect with hands on hips. Inhale deeply through the nose, hold your breath for a second or two as you form your lips into the shape of the letter O, and then exhale completely through the mouth. Repeat (for a total of two complete breaths after each rite).

Rite 1—Stand erect with arms extended straight out to the sides, palms down. Relax the shoulders and raise the arms to be in line with the shoulders. Spin in place in a clockwise direction, as fast as you can without losing control. To prevent dizziness as you spin, focus your vision on a single point straight ahead. Continue to focus on the point until it leaves your field of vision, and then focus on another point. If you become dizzy, slow down or stop. Start with just a few spins and work up to 21 revolutions.

Rite 2—Lie flat on the floor, face up with arms fully extended along sides, palms on floor, and fingers together. Raise the head from the floor, tucking the chin to the chest. As you do this, lift the legs (with the knees straight) into a vertical position. Then slowly lower both the head and the legs (keeping the knees straight) to the floor. Breathing through the nose, inhale deeply as you lift the legs, hold your breath while legs are vertical, and exhale completely as you lower the legs. Work up to 21 repetitions.

Rite 3—Kneel on the floor with the body erect, toes flexed, and hands on the back of the thighs just under the buttocks. Tilt the head and neck forward, tucking the chin to the chest. Then tilt the head and neck backward, arching the spine backward, and look upward. After arching, return to the original position. Breathing through the nose, inhale deeply as you arch the spine, hold your breath while the back is arched, and exhale completely as you return to an erect position. Work up to 21 repetitions.

Rite 4—Sit on the floor with legs extended, body erect, feet flexed and a little less than shoulder-width apart, palms flat on floor next to the hips, and fingers pointed toward feet. Tuck the chin to the chest, and then tilt the head backward as far as it will comfortably go. At the same time, bend the knees and push up to a "tabletop" position with the arms straight. Let the head fall back gently. The trunk of the body will be in a straight line, with the thighs horizontal to the floor. Tense every muscle in the body. Relax the muscles as you return to the original sitting position. Breathing through the nose, inhale deeply as you raise up, hold your breath as you tense the muscles, and exhale completely as you come down. Work up to 21 repetitions.

Rite 5—Begin face-down on all fours with your body straight, toes flexed, palms on floor, and weight distributed evenly between the palms and the balls of feet (similar to a pushup position). The hands and feet should remain in the same position throughout this rite. Start with arms perpendicular to the floor and spine arched downward, with the body in a sagging position. Slowly lift the buttocks toward the sky with the back flat, lowering the head so the body makes an inverted V. Tuck the chin to the chest. Pause, then lower the buttocks while pressing palms into the floor until legs are parallel to the ground, moving the chest out and shoulders back. Breathing through the nose, inhale deeply as you raise the body, hold your breath while in the V position, and exhale completely as you come down. Work up to 21 repetitions.

Rite 6—Stand erect and inhale through the nose. Exhale through the mouth as you bend from the waist, placing hands on knees. Expel the last bit of air from the lungs, and without taking in a new breath, return to an erect position. Place hands on hips with fingers to the front, and suck in the abdomen as much as possible. When you must take a breath, inhale through the nose and exhale through the mouth as you drop your arms down to your sides to relax. Take in several normal breaths through the nose and mouth before beginning again. Work up to three repetitions.

Relaxation—After completing the rites, spend at least five minutes in a relaxation pose. Lie flat on the floor, face up, with palms facing upward, and arms and legs extended but relaxed. Close your eyes and completely relax all the muscles in your body. Breathe deeply and easily through the nose, clearing your mind of extraneous thoughts. The relaxation period enables your body and mind to release any tension and allows the energy centers to come into balance.

The Energy Centers

The nonphysical energy centers associated with the physical body are commonly referred to as chakras (*chakra* is the Sanskrit word for *wheel*). The most valid information I have found about the energy centers is from an unusual source: an "energy personality essence no longer physically focused" (in common terms, a spirit) named Elias who speaks through a woman named Mary Ennis.[27] In an action similar to what is popularly called channeling, Ennis enters into a trance state and allows Elias to project through her. His intention is to deliver information with the least possible amount of distortion. Of the vast quantity and variety of metaphysical teachings I have studied over the years, I have found Elias's information to be the most accurate and reliable. Because so much distorted information has been offered about the chakras, Elias prefers the term *energy center*.

The information presented here about the energy centers is taken directly from the Elias session transcripts. Those familiar with the chakras will notice I included one you may never have heard of before: the pink energy center located in the upper chest, between the heart and throat. According to Elias, this is a new energy center we have developed to aid in movement within other energy centers and to promote healing and psychic activity.

In addition to the eight energy centers covered below, Elias mentions three others above the purple energy center. These energy centers (their colors are white, black, and magenta) are involved in connecting to other areas of consciousness and bringing communications from these areas into physical focus. Information about the functions of these three energy centers is beyond the scope of this book, so details about them are not included here.

Red—Located in the base of the spine. Radiates down. Governs the feet, legs, large intestine, nervous system, spine, teeth, bones, and male and female organs. Associated with grounding, sleep, and meditation. Supports the immune system in conjunction with the green and yellow energy centers. The essence of physical manifestation, this energy center holds great power. Vibrates to the tone *lo* (pronounced "low").

Orange—Located in the genitals. Radiates out. Governs the reproductive organs, kidneys, bladder, adrenal glands, skin, and bodily fluids except blood. Associated with sexual orientation and desire, life giving, and parenting. Vibrates to the tone *mu* (pronounced "moo").

Yellow—Located in the stomach. Radiates out and up. Governs the stomach, gall bladder, liver, small intestine, and pancreas. Associated with breathing (diaphragmatic), singing, all emotions, and detachment. Supports the immune system in conjunction with the red and green energy centers. Vibrates to the tone *wah* (pronounced "waw").

Green—Located in the heart. Radiates up. Governs the blood, circulatory system, heart, hands, arms, lungs, and respiratory system. Associated with the sense of touch, healing, emotion of love (transcendent), bravery, and assertiveness. Supports the immune system in conjunction with the red and yellow energy centers. Vibrates to the tone *ti* (pronounced "tee").

Pink—Located in the upper chest between the heart and throat; it is connected with and works in conjunction with the green energy center. Radiates up in conjunction with the green energy center. Associated with healing, connection, calming, and nurturing; helpful in aiding movement within other energy centers. Allows physical incorporation of subjective actualizations and increases in psychic activity. Vibrates to the tone *si* (pronounced "see").

Blue—Located in the throat. Radiates up. Governs the vocal chords, ears, shoulders, and nervous system. Associated with hearing, communication, loyalty, energy level, outlook, and self-image. Vibrates to the tone *rai* (pronounced "ray").

Indigo—Located in the center of the head, paralleling the space between the eyes. (Traditionally known as the "third eye.") Governs the eyes, nose, ears, head, and brain. Associated with bodily expressions, energy exchange, thought, intuition, and creativity. Vibrates to the tone *whou* (pronounced "hwoo," with emphasis on the "h").

Purple—Located on the top of the head, actually centered outside the physical body. Radiates up and down. Associated with spirituality, psychic energy, and physically focused consciousness. Directs all other energy centers. Vibrates to the tone *mai* (pronounced "may").

Balancing and Aligning the Energy Centers

When all the energy centers are balanced and properly aligned, our bodies and minds function optimally. The energy centers are affected by numerous nonphysical factors including our beliefs, choices, and personal issues. The yellow energy center (associated with all emotions) is the one most commonly out of alignment. The most effective way to get an energy center back to normal is to address the underlying issues. (Fears about communication, for instance, can manifest as problems with the blue energy center.) However, practices such as visualization and *toning* (using the human voice to release tensions and restore the body to a balanced, healthy state) also can be helpful for energy center realignment and balancing. Each energy center resonates with a particular note or pitch, which varies among individuals. As a general rule, the note for the red energy center is the lowest. As you move up the body, the notes become progressively higher.

Each energy center can be visualized as a sphere rotating in a clockwise direction, with the spine as the axis. (To clarify what *clockwise* means in this context, if a person standing above you could look down and see your energy centers, he would observe the spheres rotating in a clockwise direction.) Following is an energy center visualization adapted from information given in the Elias sessions:[28]

1. Imagine the spine as a thin column of white light.

2. Start with the red energy center. While toning (aloud or mentally) the sound *lo* (low), visualize a red sphere spinning clockwise at the base of the spine.

3. As you move from one energy center to the next, visualize the lower energy centers continuing to rotate, all at the same speed.

4. Move up the body to the orange energy center. While toning *mu* (moo), visualize an orange sphere spinning clockwise on the spine at the level of the lower abdomen.

5. Move up to the yellow energy center. While toning *wah* (waw), visualize a yellow sphere spinning clockwise on the spine at the level of the stomach.

6. Move up to the green energy center. While toning *ti* (tee), visualize a green sphere spinning clockwise on the spine at the level of the heart.

7. Move up to the pink energy center. While toning *si* (see), visualize a pink sphere spinning clockwise on the spine at the level of the breastbone.

8. Move up to the blue energy center. While toning *rai* (ray), visualize a blue sphere spinning clockwise on the spine at the level of the throat.

9. Move up to the indigo energy center. While toning *whou* (hwoo), visualize an indigo sphere spinning clockwise in the center of the head at eye level.

10. Move up to the purple energy center. While toning *mai* (may), visualize a purple sphere spinning clockwise just above the top of the head.

The energy centers rotate at different speeds. As you move up the body, the rate of spin increases (red is the slowest and purple the fastest). To balance the energy centers, however, it's best to visualize them all spinning at the same rate. To increase your energy level (particularly if you've been feeling sluggish or depressed), spin the energy centers rapidly. To calm yourself and reduce anxiety, spin them more slowly.

Combining the Energy Center Visualization with the Tibetan Rites

After learning about the energy centers, I started combining the energy center balancing visualization with the practice of the Five Tibetans. Rather than simply counting from 1 to 21 repetitions when performing Rites 2, 3, 4, and 5, you can sequentially visualize each energy center and mentally tone the related sound.

The following instructions appear more confusing on paper than they are in practice. Once you follow the sequence a few times, it will become second nature. Remember to imagine each of the energy centers spinning in a clockwise direction, with your spine as the axis. (In this context, *clockwise* means that if a person standing above you could look down and see your energy centers, he would observe the spheres rotating in a clockwise direction.) As you concentrate on each successive energy center, imagine all the other energy centers continuing to spin at the same rate.

Repetition 1—Mentally tone *lo* (low) while imagining a red sphere spinning at the base of your spine.

Repetition 2—Mentally tone *mu* (moo) while imagining an orange sphere spinning in your lower abdomen.

Repetition 3—Mentally tone *wah* (waw) while imagining a yellow sphere spinning in your stomach area.

Repetition 4—Combine a visualization of both the green and pink energy centers, which work together. While mentally toning *ti* (tee), imagine a green sphere spinning in your heart area and a pink sphere spinning in your upper chest.

Repetition 5—Mentally tone *rai* (ray) while imagining a blue sphere spinning in your throat area.

Repetition 6—Mentally tone *whou* (hwoo) while imagining an indigo sphere spinning in the center of your head, just above eye level.

Repetition 7—Mentally tone *mai* (may) while imagining a purple sphere spinning just above the top of your head.

Repetitions 8 through 14—Follow the above sequence in reverse, starting with the purple energy center (described in Repetition 7) and moving down the body to the indigo, blue, pink and green, yellow, orange, and red energy centers.

Repetition 15—Start again at the red energy center (described in Repetition 1) and move up the body, concluding with the purple energy center at Repetition 21.

Study the descriptions of the various energy centers and the organs and characteristics they govern. You can use this information to develop visualization techniques tailored to your individual needs.

9

Personal Care Without a Product Line

o o o o o o o o o o o o o o o o o o o o o o o o o o o o o o
"Anyone who keeps the ability to see beauty never grows old."

—Franz Kafka

Skin Care

My philosophy for personal care and beauty routines is to do the least you can to look the best you can, both short-and long-term. Spend your time and money on the practices and products that have a significant positive effect, and eliminate the rest.

In my experience, complicated and expensive skin care routines have not lived up to their claims. I still try new products occasionally, but haven't found any that have made a dramatic difference in my skin. Rather than spending a fortune on the latest "miracle" cream, start reading labels to find products that don't contain ingredients likely to be irritating. Some of the more common chemicals to avoid are sodium lauryl or laureth sulfates, ammonium lauryl or laureth sulfates, and sulfonates (detergents present in many skin cleansers, liquid soaps, shampoos, and toothpastes). These chemicals dehydrate the skin, sometimes severely. The best option for cleansing both skin and hair is a shampoo or liquid cleanser without these ingredients. (Natural foods stores carry this type of product.) Also it's best to reject products that blatantly claim to be anti-aging or wrinkle reducing. Every time you see the label, it will make you think you *need* to use something to fight aging and wrinkles.

My skin care routine is simple. First I cleanse my face with cool water and the same mild cleanser I use on my hair and body. After rinsing thoroughly, I apply moisturizer around my eyes and on any dry areas. In the morning I apply sunscreen to my face, neck, and hands.

A good way to exfoliate the skin (remove the top layer of dead cells) is with used herbal tea bags. After brewing the tea, place the tea bags in a plastic bag for later use. Cotton washcloths also can be used for exfoliation, as well as for other grooming needs. To cleanse the face and body, apply a small amount of shampoo or liquid cleanser to the cloth and use it to gently cleanse the skin (don't scrub). After bathing, a wet washcloth can be used to push back the cuticles on hands and feet. Launder washcloths frequently, since wet washcloths can harbor bacteria.

Facial Tapping

Facial tapping is a technique for stimulating acupressure points and improving circulation. I first started using it when I was applying a moisturizer and felt compelled to start tapping briskly all over my face and head with the tips of my fingers. I tapped for a couple of minutes and observed that my skin looked firmer and more vibrant. After a few weeks of tapping twice a day, the effects were even more noticeable. Several months later, I discovered that my facial tapping method is similar to *tapotement,* a massage technique that involves using the fingertips to lightly tap areas of the face or body.

The instructions for facial tapping are simple. With the fingertips (not the nails) of both hands, tap firmly enough to feel a "bounce," but not hard enough to cause pain. Tap all over the face and head for about two minutes. Perform facial tapping once a day; right after cleansing and moisturizing is a convenient time.

Following is a procedure you may want to use. There is no magic to this particular sequence; the best method is to follow your own instincts and tap where (and for how long) it feels right. Sometimes you will feel inclined to tap longer in a particular location, or you may feel like skipping a certain area altogether. As with nutrition and rest, be sensitive to the way your body feels at any given time.

1. Tap the tops of the cheekbones, moving outward and upward toward the temples.
2. Tap inward to the forehead, just above the eyebrows.

3. Tap along the brow bone, starting from the inner corner and moving in a circle around the eye socket, ending up at the nose bridge (avoid the eyeballs).
4. Tap lightly down the nose and on its sides.
5. Tap across the cheeks and out to the sides of the lower face.
6. Tap down to the lower jaw, along the jawbone, and inward to the chin.
7. Tap the chin and all around the mouth.
8. Pull the lips gently over the teeth, and tap the lips.
9. With hand flat and fingers together, tap under the chin.
10. Move up to the center of the forehead, and tap outward and upward to the head.
11. Tap along the hairline and move outward and back, tapping all over the head and the back of the neck.

You can add an extra step to help stimulate the thymus gland (the master gland of the immune system), which is located behind the breastbone. Using the knuckles or fingertips of one hand, tap about 20 times in the middle of the upper chest, about four fingers' width below the V-shaped notch at the bottom of the neck. If you are ill or feel your immune system needs a boost, tap this area for a longer time. The thymus tap can be repeated several times a day.

Instead of (or in addition to) facial tapping, you might want to try acupressure to help tone and firm facial contours and reduce wrinkles. The book *Body Reflexology* contains complete instructions and diagrams for performing an "acupressure face-lift."[29]

Sun Exposure

The issue of sun exposure and its effect on skin is paradoxical. From one perspective, the sun is necessary for life and health; how could it be harmful to us? Nevertheless, a quick look around at the complexions of most people indicates that sun exposure causes damage to unprotected skin. More accurately, it shows that our culture has a strong *belief* that sun exposure damages skin; therefore it does. (There are, however, individuals who do not align with this belief and regularly expose their unprotected skin to the sun without adverse effects.)

Ironically, some of the skin damage blamed on sunlight may be due to exposure to fluorescent lighting, which can adversely affect the skin.

As with beliefs about toxic substances, the belief that exposure to ultraviolet light (both from natural and artificial sources) causes damage to unprotected skin is deeply ingrained in our culture. This is an area where I find it easier to go along with what I believe rather than try to convince myself otherwise. In my experience, consistent use of nonchemical sunscreens for several years has maintained—even improved—the condition and appearance of my skin.

Although the sun apparently does cause detrimental changes in unprotected skin, *some* direct sun exposure is beneficial and necessary for our health. The optimal areas for direct exposure may be the backs of the knees and insides of the elbows, where the skin is thin and blood vessels are close to the surface. The face, neck, and hands usually have been overexposed to the sun for so many years that I don't recommend leaving them unprotected. A better option is to periodically get some direct sun exposure on the legs and/or arms for at least a few minutes a day.

For optimum health, we also need to be exposed to the full spectrum of natural light through our eyes.[30] Corrective lenses and window glass block some of these rays. For those who spend most of the day indoors, wearing ultraviolet-blocking sunglasses every time they're in direct sunlight is probably not the best practice. When dark glasses are worn, the pupils dilate to adjust to the darkness. When the glasses are removed, the eye is suddenly exposed to bright light when it is least able to deal with it. Indoor types might do well to limit the use of sunglasses to times when they are in intense sunlight for an extended period of time or are driving in bright sunshine. A good guideline to follow is that if you need to squint due to the sun's brightness or glare, then shade your eyes with a hat, visor, or sunglasses.

Selecting a Sunscreen

The best sunscreens have micronized (ground into tiny particles) zinc oxide as the active ingredient, with no added chemical sunscreens. Zinc oxide blocks the broadest spectrum of ultraviolet A (UVA) and ultraviolet B (UVB) rays, as well as infrared rays, which also may damage the skin. UVB rays have their greatest effect on the epidermis (the outer, protective layer of the skin) and are mostly responsible for burning, tanning, hyperpigmentation (dark spots), and basal cell carcinoma (the most common and least serious form of skin cancer). UVA rays are longer and penetrate more deeply, causing damage to the dermis (the lower, connective tissue layer of the skin) that ultimately can result in loss of elasticity and other changes associated with aging. Another reason I prefer zinc oxide is that it doesn't have the irritation potential of chemical sunscreens. When applied to the skin, products with micronized zinc oxide do not have the stark white look characteristic of the original zinc oxide sunscreens.

Another commonly used natural (mineral) sunscreen is titanium dioxide, which is the active ingredient in many sunscreens labeled *nonchemical*. However, titanium dioxide blocks only part of the spectrum of UVA rays, so it isn't as effective as zinc oxide. It also is more visible (ashy-looking) on the skin. In addition, I prefer zinc because it is more natural to the body than titanium (zinc is an essential nutrient).

Contrary to popular belief, the Sun Protection Factor (SPF) of a sunscreen product is not of paramount importance. SPF measures only the sunscreen's ability to block UVB (not UVA) rays. Products with micronized zinc oxide as the only sunscreen ingredient usually have an SPF of 15 or less, yet they provide substantially more UVA protection than many of the chemical-containing sunscreens that are labeled SPF 30 or higher. Most products with a very high SPF are full of potentially irritating chemical sunscreens. When I used chemical sunscreens in the past, I noticed that many of them caused my skin to feel very irritated when it was exposed to sunlight, to the point that I had to wash off the product. The much-touted UVA sunscreen avobenzone (Parsol 1789) breaks down rapidly when exposed to ultraviolet light—it can lose most of its potency in as little as one hour of sun exposure. For these reasons, I avoid products that contain chemical sunscreens.

My preference is for sunscreens that contain at least 10 percent micronized zinc oxide, no chemical sunscreen ingredients, and no titanium dioxide. Unfortunately, sunscreens with zinc oxide as the only active ingredient are not yet widely available. As of this writing, the only company I know of that offers this type of product is BirchTrees, Inc. Their Daily Guard Sun Screen contains 15 percent micronized zinc oxide and has an SPF of 15. The product can be ordered directly from the company by mail at BirchTrees Inc., 851 S.E. Monterey Commons Boulevard, Stuart, Florida 34996 USA; by phone at 772-283-1315 or 1-888-440-1315 (toll-free); or online at *www.birchtrees.com*.

For sun protection for lips, natural foods stores carry lip balms made of plant oils and waxes that contain micronized zinc oxide and chemical sunscreens. (Two companies that offer this type of product are All Terrain and Ecco Bella.) If you wear lip color, you can apply a light layer of micronized zinc oxide sunscreen to your lips before applying the lip color. A full-coverage lipstick provides some sun protection even if it doesn't contain sunscreen.

Hair Care

As with skin cleansers, avoid shampoos that contain sulfates or sulfonates. If you use a shampoo that doesn't contain these drying chemicals, you may not even need a hair conditioner. You can condition any dry areas by applying a few drops of natural oil (such as jojoba, almond, avocado, or apricot) or a very small amount of a skin balm made from natural oils. The oil or balm can be applied to damp or dry hair. For deep conditioning, apply a larger amount of oil before you wash your hair, and leave it on for at least 10 minutes. Enough oil will remain after shampooing to condition the hair in a natural way. Natural oils and skins balms are sold in natural foods stores and some pharmacies.

Blow dryers and other heated appliances can damage hair, especially if used frequently. Blow dryers also expose the user to a high level of electromagnetic frequencies, which isn't a particularly good thing to blast your brain with. Try drying your hair naturally instead. Remove excess moisture by pressing gently with a towel. Comb out the tangles, apply a little oil or balm to dry areas, arrange your hair the way you like it, and let it air-dry the rest of the way.

Acupressure methods can also benefit the hair and scalp. A technique called *nail buffing* can help stimulate hair growth on the head. To perform nail buffing, place the four fingernails of one hand (leave out the thumb) against the four fingernails of the other hand and rub them together briskly for at least 60 seconds. In addition to enhancing the hair, nail buffing is said to increase energy levels throughout the body.[31]

Dental Care

The only dental care products truly necessary for most people are dental floss and a toothbrush with soft, end-rounded, polished bristles. The use of toothpicks and dental stimulators also helps clean the teeth and stimulate the gums. Another way to remove plaque and stimulate gum circulation is to massage the gums with your index finger wrapped in a clean, wet washcloth.

If you use toothpaste, choose a formula that is low in abrasion and does not contain fluoride. Currently there's a great deal of controversy about the practice of adding fluoride to public water supplies and dental products. Excessive intake of fluoride can damage developing teeth (a condition known as *dental fluorosis*) and adversely affect the bones and other body systems. Keep in mind that fluoride is present not only in dental products and drinking water, but also in soft drinks, juices, and canned and frozen foods.

Dentists are the only health professionals I visit on a regular basis. However, I've met several people with healthy teeth and gums who haven't been to a dentist in years. If you use dental services, it's imperative to find a dentist that is highly skilled and knowledgeable about overall health. Inappropriate dental work can cause a myriad of health problems throughout the body. When choosing a dentist, I immediately rule out those that still use amalgam (silver) fillings, even if they offer alternatives. Amalgam contains mercury, and anyone who would put a toxic substance like mercury into a person's mouth cannot be trusted with health-related decisions. My preference is to have no metal at all in my mouth. Metals in dental restorations (including precious metals like gold and platinum) can affect the body's energy field. Also I favor dentists with a conservative "less is more" approach to dental work in general. For instance, a small cavity that is no longer actively decaying may not need to be drilled and filled.

Like the rest of your body, teeth and gums are affected by your beliefs and intentions. I know of at least two cases in which individuals were told they needed dental work, but they corrected the problems themselves with their intention and belief they could do so. They went back to the dentist a few months later and were told they no longer needed the previously recommended procedures. This is yet another area in which we are limited only by our beliefs of what is possible. Teeth are living structures that can regenerate.

Vision Care

In the late 1800s and early 1900s, ophthalmologist Dr. William H. Bates developed techniques for improving eyesight that helped eliminate the need for corrective lenses in many individuals. His method was so successful that it is still being used and taught all over the world, and there are numerous books based on his ideas. Bates's own book (which is still in print) is called *The Bates Method for Better Eyesight Without Glasses*.[32] To find out more about the Bates Method, contact the Bates Association for Vision Education (mailing address: Savoy Court Hotel, 11-15 Cavendish Place, Eastbourne, East Sussex, United Kingdom BN21 3EJ) or refer to their website, *www.seeing.org*.

An eye relaxation technique Bates recommended for everyone is called *palming*. To perform palming, cup your hands and place them over your closed eyes without putting any pressure on the eyeballs. Relax the eye muscles, and preferably the rest of your body as well. The aim is to allow as little light as possible to enter the eye, so a darkened room is ideal. If you are lying down in a lighted room, put a towel or cloth over your hands to block out more light. Palming at least once a day for five minutes or more is ideal (a good time is right before you go to sleep at night). Alternatively, you can take numerous mini-breaks throughout the day by palming for one minute or less.

Another way to help maintain acute vision is to avoid staring rigidly in the same position for an extended period of time. Move your eyes and head regularly. When you are reading, doing paperwork, or using a computer, look up every few minutes and briefly focus on something far away. Don't stare or strain; simply focus on the point for a moment or two. (For instance, read the title of a book on a shelf across the room.) Take short breaks from your work by alternately looking at objects that are far away, very close, and a medium distance from you.

Certain nutrients can help maintain vision and improve eye health. Lutein and zeaxanthin (antioxidants in the carotenoid family) are particularly good for the eyes. Both nutrients are present in high concentrations in kale, spinach, and other dark green leafy vegetables. Bilberries contain high levels of lutein.

Plastic Surgery

Ideally, at some point we will have our beliefs in alignment with our desires and therefore won't manifest signs of age-related degeneration. Presently, that's obviously not the case. Like other medical treatments, plastic surgery can be used as a tool to make changes on a physical level that we haven't yet been able to create internally. This view is different from the approach of desperately attempting to hold onto one's youth by trying every new cosmetic procedure reported in the latest magazines. If you believe age-related degeneration is inevitable and are attempting to do everything possible to stave it off, then plastic surgery (like any other anti-aging technique) will be a stopgap measure at best. If you choose to have plastic surgery, following are some points to keep in mind:

- Choose an excellent surgeon, preferably one with extensive experience in performing the procedure(s) you are interested in. Ask to see before-and-after pictures, and if possible, talk to a couple of former patients. Above all, follow your intuition and feelings about whether a particular doctor is right for you. Good credentials and references are important, but don't let these override your own instincts.

- The three most important words in plastic surgery are: *communication, communication, communication.* It is of the utmost importance to clearly communicate your desired results to your doctor, and for the doctor to thoroughly explain what he or she thinks can be accomplished. In addition, make sure you understand any possible complications and what to expect during the recovery period (including the activity restrictions you will need to follow).

- Be cautious about having any substance injected or implanted into your face or body. Before making a decision to undergo this type of procedure, obtain as much information about the substance as you can. New compounds are continually being developed, and sometimes these materials have adverse affects that don't become apparent until years after the procedure.

- Know when to quit. Sometimes when an individual has one or two cosmetic procedures and is happy with the result, he or she continues to have more and more plastic surgery. After a certain point, the person starts to look unnatural, possibly even ghoulish. The most successful cosmetic operations leave patients looking like themselves, only better.

PART IV
Additional Areas

10

Streamlining and Simplifying

o o o o o o o o o o o o o o o o o o o o o o o o o o o o o o o
"Our life is frittered away by detail…Simplify, simplify!"

—*Henry David Thoreau*[33]

Old Stuff Leads to Old Folks

Could hanging on to old stuff possibly have anything to do with aging? Surprisingly, it does. Not letting go of physical objects is a reflection of our unwillingness to release old emotional issues and outworn ideas. When we retain these things in our energy field, they affect the physical body. If we want our bodies to start fresh with optimally functioning, undamaged cells, then we must learn to start fresh and release everything we are holding onto that no longer serves us.

Many people keep too much stuff largely out of fear—fear that they will need it in the future, or for some other reason will regret getting rid it. Yet having too many possessions can sap your life force energy. There's a part of your life force in everything you own, as well as in all your commitments. Do you really want your energy to be dissipated into three closets full of clothes, two motor vehicles, and 23 appliances?

In modern society, we've learned not to trust ourselves and to rely on outside means of verification instead. Many of our products (medications, nutritional supplements, and cosmetics) are props we've come to believe we need to use to maintain our physical bodies. Clocks, thermometers, scales, and other measurement and monitoring systems have taken the place of our own senses. When we learn to rely more on our innate capabilities, we may find we don't need so many material things.

Clutter and Excess Weight

Can clutter make you fat? As with aging, having too much stuff is related to being overweight. In both cases, a person has taken on (or in) more than they need or can use. Part of the reason so many people are overweight may be that they are unwilling or afraid to let go of things they no longer need. Just as their closets, bureaus, and basements are stuffed with more possessions than they require, their body's storage areas are overfilled as well. When you alter your attitude and habits so that you acquire and use only the items you need, you can apply this new awareness to your food choices and eating habits as well. Over time, without dieting, you'll find that your weight readjusts to a healthier level.

Streamlining Suggestions

Following are a few ideas for simplifying and streamlining:

- The basics of streamlining are to eliminate, simplify, and organize—in that order. When you implement organizing systems and methods, make them as simple as possible.

- Streamlining doesn't mean going back to basics and ignoring modern advances. Keep up with technological developments, new products, and fashion trends, but incorporate only those that appeal to you. When you add something new, dispose of the old version (don't just stuff it in the back of a closet).

- Consciously choose the objects, relationships, and commitments you want in your life. Eliminate anything that no longer is (or never was) important to you, including possessions, activities, and relationships. If you pare down in most areas, you will have more resources for the things that are most important and enjoyable to you now.

- An interest, hobby, or activity you enjoyed in the past may not be something you want to continue. Be honest with yourself, and let it go. Sell or donate the equipment, collection, or other paraphernalia to someone who will benefit from it as you once did. Divesting yourself of what is no longer useful creates room in your life (both literally and figuratively) for new interests. Keep things (books, money, ideas) in circulation; don't hoard or hang onto what you no longer need.

- Get rid of *anything* that makes you feel bad when you look at or think about it. There is a physical, electromagnetic reality to the associations we make with objects. Owning an object connects you to things you might not want to be connected to, such as a former spouse or a job you disliked. A ring from an old boyfriend doesn't just remind you of him; it energetically links you to him.

- Before you buy an item, consider not just if it will serve your needs and is a reasonable price, but how much complication it will create in your life. Think about the complications that can accompany owning just one appliance or electronic device: you have to file the instructions, warranty, and receipt; purchase batteries, bulbs, or special cleaning products; and clean, repair, and possibly insure the item. Think about whether or not the function it serves in your life is important enough to outweigh the complications it creates.

- If you don't already use the Internet, consider doing so—it's a great streamlining tool. Having access to information in electronic form makes it unnecessary to keep so many reference books, telephone directories, catalogs, reports, articles, letters, and other paper items. Just think of all the trees that can be saved!

Use It or Lose It

For streamlining your living spaces, follow the advice of nineteenth century poet and decorator William Morris: "Have nothing in your houses that you do not know to be useful or believe to be beautiful."

Decluttering is most effective when done in stages. First, go through the items in a particular category, remove the ones you know you should get rid of, and make decisions on the "maybes." After you have finished evaluating all your possessions and disposing of the excess (a process that may take days, weeks, or months), take a break and enjoy the feelings of pride, satisfaction, and freedom you'll have as a result of your efforts. When you feel like cleaning up again (and you will—decluttering can become addictive), go back to the first areas you decluttered and reevaluate the items you kept. It's likely you will identify additional items you no longer want to keep. Over time, review all the areas you decluttered. You'll be surprised at how much more you can dispose of.

To prepare for the decluttering process, you'll need six large containers such as boxes, bags, or wastebaskets. You will use these containers for items to be: (1) thrown away, (2) donated to charity, (3) given or returned to other people, (4) cleaned or repaired, (5) moved to another location, and (6) decided on later. Make decisions as you go along, but if you're really stumped about something, put it in the sixth container rather than wasting a lot of time on it. When evaluating your possessions, ask yourself:

- How do I feel about this item?
- How often do I use it?
- Do I have other items that serve the same purpose?
- If it were lost or destroyed, would I buy another one?
- If it isn't replaceable, would I really miss it or be relieved that it was gone?
- What is the worst thing that could happen if I needed this item and didn't have it?

First pare down to the things you really use, and then evaluate those to see if you could manage with fewer items. For example, you may have five shampoos and nine different types of ink pens. You might use each of them occasionally, but do you really need all those variations? If you want to keep more than one of a certain item, set a quantity limit. For example, allow yourself a maximum of four types of ink pens, two pairs of athletic shoes, and so forth. If you want to add another, eliminate one of the old ones.

For things you know you should get rid of but can't bring yourself to part with just yet, use the following method: Pack the items in boxes or bags and put them in a storage area, preferably where you won't see them often. On your calendar, mark a date three months in the future. When the day of reckoning arrives, either go through the boxes again or (if you're brave) dispose of them without looking at the contents. If you haven't needed something in three months, you can live without it. When you finally dispose of something you've been mulling over, you are free from having to make that decision ever again. Each time you think about an item and decide not to get rid of it, you know you'll have to evaluate it again in the future.

Some people feel they are being wasteful if they dispose of an item that's still in good condition. Yet if you don't really need something that could be used by others, it's more wasteful to keep it than to give it away. Many charitable organizations accept donations of useful items and will give you a receipt for income tax documentation. If you don't already know of such an organization, look under the Social Services listing in the Yellow Pages. Some charities have a pickup service that will come to your home, which makes it easy to donate furniture and larger items.

Managing New Purchases

When decluttering, your motto should be *If in doubt, throw it out.* When shopping, however, if in doubt, leave it out (of the shopping cart). As with eating, it's best not to get in the habit of using shopping (whether at malls, boutiques, or yard sales) as a purely recreational activity. I can imagine the shopping mall planners saying, "If we build them, they will spend." If you go, you will buy.

To avoid recluttering your newly decluttered areas, be judicious about acquiring additional items. Before making a decision to purchase something, ask yourself the following questions:

- How will owning this improve my life?
- Do I already have something that serves the same purpose? If so, am I willing to get rid of the old one?
- Do I truly want this item, or am I responding to advertisements, other people's expectations, or the force of habit?
- Would I be interested in buying this item if it wasn't on sale?
- Is the item described as a *collectible* or *collector's item*? It may not say so in the dictionary, but these terms are synonyms for clutter.
- Where will I put it, and how much space will it take up?
- What type of maintenance, cleaning, and/or replaceable parts does this item require?
- Can the item (and its parts or service) be acquired only from special stores, catalogs, or vendors? If I move to a different area, will there be a problem obtaining parts or service?
- Can I borrow or rent this item instead of buying it?

With clothing and fashion accessories, avoid buying those that: (1) are uncomfortable or don't fit well; (2) will be difficult or expensive to maintain, such as clothing that must be ironed, hand washed, or dry cleaned frequently; (3) don't coordinate with your current wardrobe and therefore will require other purchases; (4) are very similar to items you already own (unless you plan to get rid of one of the old ones).

Unless you truly need or want something, don't accept it just because someone offers it to you for free. You probably already know that renting space in a storage facility is expensive, but the space used for storing things in your home also costs money (a portion of your mortgage or rent). The next time you're tempted to acquire something you don't need just because it's offered for free or at a bargain price, think about how much it will cost you to store it. Think about what it's costing you to store the unnecessary stuff you already have.

Your Stuff and Your Identity

Remember that you are more than just what you *own* (material possessions) and what you *do* (to earn a living). If you lost your job and your savings, your house burned down, and all your belongings were destroyed, would you feel you had lost your identity? Perhaps one of the reasons many people are so afraid of dying is that they know they won't be able take any of their stuff with them, and they don't know who they would be without it. Your identity is intrinsic to your being; it doesn't depend upon external factors or possessions.

11

The Ultimate Taboo

○ ○
"Life is eternal; and love is immortal; and death is only a horizon; and a horizon is nothing save the limit of our sight."

—Rossiter W. Raymond

The Longevity Question

With even a cursory look at this book, it's apparent that I don't believe age-related degeneration is inevitable. Unlike many of those in the anti-aging camp, however, I have no interest in promoting the idea of physical immortality or even extreme longevity. It's likely that humans could routinely live well over 100 years if they wanted to do so and believed it was possible, but physical mortality was one of the "ground rules" when we chose to be born into this world. If you truly believe that more exists than what we experience in this physical dimension, then what's the point of striving for physical immortality anyway? Personally I've never had a desire for extreme longevity, and since childhood have known I won't reach an advanced age. When I've had close calls in which I could easily have been killed or seriously injured, afterwards I felt a great appreciation—almost a feeling of euphoria—for being alive and healthy, which is something I take for granted most of the time. Yet I'm not particularly afraid of death (except for fears about dying in a horrible or painful way), and I have no doubt that we continue to exist afterward.

Occasionally it has been suggested that perhaps I don't want to live to an old age so I can avoid the degeneration most people believe is inevitable, but that isn't the reason. Even with a perennially youthful body and brain (which is something we all have the ability to create), I still would choose not to live to an advanced age. At some point well before the 100-year mark, I expect I'll feel I've had enough experience in this realm and will want to move on. As my friend John put it, "I imagine death to be somewhat like coming home from a long trip. You enjoyed the trip, but are really glad to be back home." If our cultural beliefs about death were more in line with what truly happens, I suspect more people would feel this way.

An Alternative View of Death

Ironically, with the many authentic phenomena that our mainstream culture fails to acknowledge (telepathy, clairvoyance, energy healing, and so forth), some things almost universally accepted as genuine are actually invalid. Prominent among these false concepts is our idea of death: the belief that a conscious personality can truly cease to exist. The human body can be destroyed, but consciousness cannot be extinguished—it merely changes form. If we truly understood this concept, we would be much more accepting of a person's choice to pass on. Yes, it is a *choice*: every individual who leaves physical life has chosen to do so, although they may not be consciously paying attention to this choice.

In our culture, death is viewed not as a choice, but as a failure: the doctors failed to save the patient and the patient failed to survive. How often have you heard people say things like, "He lost his battle with cancer"? In many cases, individuals who are ready to die will prolong their pain and suffering because they know their loved ones aren't ready to let go. It would serve us well to learn to accept death as a natural part of life rather than viewing it as something to be feared and conquered. Some individuals do have this attitude. When they feel it is time to move on from this world, they simply sit down, go into a meditative state, and quietly leave their body. This practice is common enough among advanced yoga masters in India that there's even a word for it: *mahasamadhi*. This apparent "voluntary death" is almost incomprehensible to many Westerners, but to me it seems a much better choice than suffering with illness or trauma.

Given our cultural attitudes about death, the following idea may seem appalling, but I'm suggesting it anyway. Instead of trying to keep people alive at all costs, we could accept that we are going to die and plan for it—much like the way employees give notice before they leave a job, and their coworkers arrange a going-away celebration. As it's usually done now, friends and family get together only after their loved one has passed on. In cases where a person knows she has a limited amount of time left, it would make more sense to have everyone get together while she is still alive. Rather than just reminiscing about the person after she's passed on, they could enjoy visiting with her while she's still here.

The Mystery of Life After Death

Many people fear death largely because they don't know what to expect when it occurs. Regardless of our religious or philosophical beliefs, most of us feel pretty clueless about what happens to people when they leave this realm. I expect that dying will be a lot like waking up from a dream: I will experience much greater clarity and be relieved to find that the problems and situations I've been struggling with aren't "real." The idea that nothing exists beyond this physical life is as ludicrous to me as the idea that nothing exists outside of the building I'm in now. I may not be able to physically see anything else at the moment, but that doesn't mean it isn't there.

The numerous accounts of near-death experiences support the fact that there is life after death, but they don't necessarily provide an accurate description of what may happen to each of us when we pass on. I believe near-death experiences are very real; they aren't hallucinations any more than our daily waking life is a hallucination. However, these experiences are heavily influenced by a person's beliefs and expectations about what happens after death. A Christian may see angels or Jesus Christ, for instance, while a Hindu may encounter the god Brahma or the goddess Lakshmi. Near-death experiences differ from actual death in a fundamental way: the person ultimately returns to our physical reality. I consider near-death experiences to be like field trips to another realm. The first few minutes after death don't reveal what the afterlife is truly like any more than the first few minutes after birth give an accurate idea of what a human's physical life will be like.

After many years of metaphysical study, I've come to believe that what people experience after physical death is based upon the beliefs they hold in life. Therefore, individuals' after-death experiences can vary greatly. While I don't think there is a heaven or hell as depicted in religious belief systems, someone who believes in the existence of heaven can actually create such a place, complete with winged angels floating on clouds. A person with similar beliefs who feels he has lived an evil life may create a fiery hell populated with suffering sinners and pitchfork-wielding devils. Fortunately these creations are only temporary; eventually the person moves past these beliefs.

Messages from those who have passed on (communicated through professional mediums and numerous personal accounts) almost overwhelmingly indicate that people are happier in the afterlife than they were in their physical lives. I once visited a psychic reader who knew immediately (without my giving her any information) that one of my relatives had died within the past month.

She told me she sensed that the woman was pointing to her head and chest (the areas where she'd had cancer) and saying, "If I had known how it would be here [in the afterlife], I wouldn't have fought [death] so hard." In two other instances, friends have told me of experiences in which they were extremely distraught over a loved one's passing, and the departed person actually paid them a visit. In neither case did the person speak, but they looked so joyful and radiant that there was no doubt they were happy in their new environment.

Continuing Communication

Many people who suspend their disbelief in the possibility of communication with individuals who have departed this realm find they can continue the relationship, albeit in an altered form. Such communication can be accomplished through another person (a medium), but there are other methods as well. Direct interaction with those "on the other side" may occur in dreams and also can be achieved through intention and focus while in a relaxed, meditative state. Simply opening yourself to these types of experiences (and paying attention throughout the day) will allow you to notice communications that may come in subtle ways. For instance, you may be thinking about the person, wondering how he is doing in his new environment, and then you turn on the radio and hear a song that gives you the answer. Communications of this type can come from virtually any source: people, animals, birds, plants, books, music, movies, and television, in addition to your own feelings and impressions.

The potential for communication after physical death can perhaps best be illustrated by an analogy. A woman I know named Anne, well loved by her many friends and family members, passed on after struggling with cancer for several years. She maintained her optimistic disposition even in the worst of times, and she is deeply missed by her loved ones. Rather than believing that Anne is "dead and gone," I view the situation much as if she simply relocated from her home in Virginia to a far-away country. She loved being near her family and friends, but the climate and conditions in Virginia did not agree with her anymore. In her new home, she has completely regained her health and feels good again. It's been many years since Anne visited the place, so there is much for her to explore in that beautiful country, as well as many old friends whom she hasn't seen in a long time.

While Anne will miss her loved ones in the United States (and it will be quite awhile before she sees most of them face-to-face again), they can keep in touch with her via letters, telephone calls, electronic mail, and other means of communication. In order to do this, however, her friends and family must acknowledge that (1) Anne is still alive, and (2) it is possible to communicate with her. They may not be able to establish communication immediately; it may take some time for Anne to get her bearings in her new home. Also, the view from her new vantage point will be much broader. Her awareness will encompass a great deal more than it did prior to her passing; therefore her attention is likely to be focused in areas other than our physical world. Eventually, however, she may make contact, especially if she senses people would like to hear from her.

In order for this system to work, however, Ann's loved ones will have to put up a mailbox, connect their telephone, or get an electronic mail account—and they need to check for messages regularly. If they don't believe Ann's personality is still alive and accessible from our physical world, then these avenues of communication will remain closed to them. The real tragedy here is not Ann's passing, but our failure to recognize the true nature of her physical death: that it is a transition rather than an ending, and that she can still be a part of our lives.

This story sounds wonderful, you may be thinking, but has anyone (other than a few famous mediums) ever accomplished this sort of thing? The answer is yes—many people have done so, including several I've known. In fact, recently I heard from a mutual friend that Anne's husband mentioned that his departed wife is still telling him what to do!

In another example, Jeanette, a friend I used to work with, communicated with her father in the dream state for several years after he passed on. On a regular basis, she had dreams in which she was talking with her father. Often he would give her helpful advice on situations she was dealing with in her life. The last year of Jeanette's father's life coincided with the first year of her son's life, and one of her father's greatest joys was spending time with the baby. It was virtually the only time he wasn't in pain from the cancer he was suffering with. One night a couple of months after his death, Jeanette was having a terrible time with the baby's incessant crying. She had gotten up numerous times to attend to her son, but nothing she did would soothe him for long. Sleep-deprived and frustrated, Jeanette was losing her ability to cope with the situation. Once again the child started screaming, so she got out of bed and went into in his room. When she walked in the door, Jeanette was dumbfounded. Not only had the baby stopped crying, he was smiling and giggling softly. Her son was looking upward and acting as if someone were standing over the crib and playing with him! The scene was eerily familiar to Jeanette. It was as if, once again, her father was standing there playing with his beloved grandson. She watched for a couple of minutes, and then returned to her room without disturbing the child. He was quiet for the rest of the night.

It often is easier for small children to communicate with the departed simply because they have not yet learned that it isn't supposed to be possible. A colleague once told me that his four-year-old daughter said she regularly talked with her departed great-grandmother. One time he saw the little girl alone in her room, apparently having a conversation with someone he couldn't see. The family had been very worried about his wife's mother, who was in the hospital recovering from surgery. The little girl came bouncing out of her room, ecstatic because her great-grandmother had just told her, "Grandma is going to be fine." And indeed she was.

Regarding intentional communication with those who have passed on, keep in mind that they may not contact us every time we want them to. After death, people don't become static and remain just as you remembered them; their awareness is much broader, and they grow and change with their new experiences. Much like a teenager who goes away to college, they may get so caught up in these experiences that they forget to "answer our calls." It doesn't mean they don't care about us; it simply means their attention is focused elsewhere. Also (to continue my earlier analogy), sometimes the telephone lines are down or there is interference from the weather. The dream state is often the easiest avenue for those who have passed on to make contact with us, as we're generally the most receptive then. The fundamental thing to remember is that when loved ones leave their physical bodies, nothing has been "lost"—they are alive as they ever were, and the connection you share with them is eternal.

A Broader Perspective

A friend of mine, Justin, once described a dream he'd had. The setting of the dream was a huge party in the afterlife. Justin was there with everyone he had ever known, everyone *they* had ever known, and so on. All the people were having a great time, talking and laughing about who had done what to whom. It was much like a cast party after a stage play, when the person who played the murderer is joyfully sharing a meal with the "victim." Both actors know that what happened in the play doesn't really make any difference. Beneath the costumes and makeup, they are good friends who care deeply about one another.

Justin's dream struck me as quite profound. It's a great illustration of the way I believe things really are, once we get past our beliefs in right-versus-wrong and good-versus-evil. In our day-to-day dramas, each of us simply plays our role. In the larger scheme of things, no one ever dies.

Afterword

From my personal experience, I advise readers not to expect sudden, dramatic changes when they start incorporating these ideas. Certainly it's possible to undergo an abrupt alteration, but with longstanding, deeply rooted beliefs, there's usually a more gradual shift. The new ideas begin infiltrating your consciousness, and the more you reinforce them, the stronger they become. The less you reinforce the old beliefs (by thinking and talking about getting old, worrying about age-associated disorders, and so forth), the sooner they fade away.

Once you recognize that something is a belief rather than an absolute truth, it gives you the freedom to choose whether or not you want to hold that belief and be subject to its "rules." When we truly realize that nearly all age-related degeneration is due to our belief in it, most of us will automatically make the choice not to align with that belief. It really is that simple.

It's best to avoid monitoring yourself for physical signs of aging or youthfulness, which tends to make you focus on (and therefore perpetuate) the characteristics you dislike. Instead, let the positive changes sneak up on you. A year from now, you may see an old photo of yourself and realize you look younger now than you did then. Perhaps you will notice that some physical problems have simply disappeared, or that your characteristic mental sharpness has returned. As your beliefs shift over time, you will find that your experience of aging differs more and more from the experiences of your contemporaries.

Applying these ideas has made a significant difference in my own experience of aging. From my early twenties to mid-thirties (when I held conventional beliefs about aging), people typically assumed I was at least five years older than my chronological age. In recent years, this trend has reversed—now, people often think I'm several years younger than my actual age. In addition, I haven't noticed any decline in physical or mental functioning, nor have I developed any age-related conditions or diseases.

In the past, when I noticed physical signs of aging in a person (myself or someone else), I thought of them as a natural consequence of getting older. Now I consider such signs to be evidence not of advancing age, but of the person's *belief* that the body degenerates with age. Viewed in that manner, physical signs of aging are helpful communications about the state of one's beliefs. Also, I no longer consider aging-related changes to be permanent, irreversible conditions that inevitably will worsen over time. I expect my body to change as my beliefs change, which means I may well start looking *younger* as the years go by.

You now have the knowledge that your existence does not have to be a downward spiral from the peak of young adulthood to a dismal old age. When you think about aging and health, above all, remember that your physical body is a manifestation of what you create through your beliefs and choices. Our DNA does not dictate our destiny—we have the power to change anything in our experience. As long as you are alive, you possess the ability to truly *live*.

"Since everything is but an apparition, perfect in being what it is, having nothing to do with good or bad, acceptance or rejection, one may well burst out in laughter."

—Longchenpa

Notes

Introduction

1. Fred Alan Wolf, Ph.D., *Taking the Quantum Leap: The New Physics for Non-Scientists* (New York, NY: Harper & Row Publishers, Perennial Library, 1989, revised edition), p. 128.

Chapter 1

2. Bruce H. Lipton, Ph.D., "The Biology of Belief" (2001), http://www.brucelipton.com.

3. Lipton.

4. Lipton.

5. Osamu Nishikaze, Ph.D., University of Hokkaido, Japan.

6. Michael Talbot, *The Holographic Universe* (New York, NY: HarperCollins Publishers, HarperPerennial, 1991), pp. 87–88.

7. Stephen Hawley Martin, *Past Fear and Doubt to Amazing Abundance: Secret Knowledge That Brought Me Self-Actualization* (Richmond, VA: The Oaklea Press, 2000), pp. 9–10.

8. Robert M. Williams, M.A., *The Missing (Piece) Peace in Your Life!* (Crestone, CO: Myrddin Corporation, Spirit 2000 Publications, 2002), pp. 115–117.

Chapter 2

9. Bob Dylan, "My Back Pages" (Special Rider Music, 1964 and 1992).

10. Talbot, pp. 98–99.

11. Peter Ragnar, *How Long Do You Choose to Live? A Question of a Lifetime* (Gatlinburg, TN: Roaring Lion Publishing, 2001).

Chapter 3

12. J. L. Glaser, J. L. Brind, J. H. Vogelman, M. J. Eisner, M. C. Dillbeck, R. K. Wallace, D. Chopra, and N. Orentreich, "Elevated serum dehydroepiandrosterone sulfate levels in practitioners of the Transcendental Meditation (TM) and TM-Sidhi programs," Journal of Behavioral Medicine, 1992, Vol. 15(4), pp. 327–341.

13. Michael Sky, *Breathing: Expanding Your Power and Energy* (Santa Fe, NM: Bear & Company Publishing, 1990).

14. Sky, pp. 69–72.

Chapter 4

15. Mary Ennis, The Elias Transcripts (held in © copyright 1995–2001 by Mary Ennis and Vicki Pendley, © copyright 2001–2004 by Mary Ennis), Elias Session 1105, June 8, 2002.

16. Jane Roberts and Robert F. Butts (Contributor), *Seth Speaks: The Eternal Validity of the Soul* (San Rafael, CA: Amber-Allen Publishing, 1994, reissue edition), p. 163, Session 546, Aug. 19, 1970.

17. Roberts and Butts, *The Nature of Personal Reality: Specific, Practical Techniques for Solving Everyday Problems and Enriching the Life You Know (A Seth Book)* (San Rafael, CA: Amber-Allen Publishing, 1994, reissue edition), p. 45, Session 617, Sept. 25, 1972.

18. Talbot, pp. 106–108.

Chapter 6

19. Louise L. Hay, *Heal Your Body: The Mental Causes for Physical Illness and the Metaphysical Way to Overcome Them* (Carlsbad, CA: Hay House, 2003, reissue edition).

20. Hay, p. 62.

21. Mildred Carter and Tammy Weber, *Body Reflexology: Healing at Your Fingertips* (Paramus, NJ: Parker Publishing Company, Reward Books, 1994, revised and updated edition).

22. Talbot, pp. 150–152.

Chapter 8

23. Peter Kelder, *Ancient Secret of the Fountain of Youth: Book 1* (Gig Harbor, WA: Harbor Press, 1998, reissue edition).

24. Christopher S. Kilham, *The Five Tibetans: Five Dynamic Exercises for Health, Energy, and Personal Power* (Rochester, VT: Inner Traditions International, Healing Arts Press, 1994).

25. Kelder, pp. 46–54.

26. Kilham, pp. 54–55.

27. Ennis, Elias Digests–Energy Centers (Body), http://www.eliasforum.org.

28. Ennis.

Chapter 9

29. Carter and Weber, pp. 296–303.

30. Jacob Liberman, O.D, Ph.D., *Light: Medicine of the Future* (Santa Fe, NM: Bear & Company Publishing, 1991), pp. 51 and 175–177.

31. Carter and Weber, pp. 188–190.

32. William H. Bates, M.D., *The Bates Method for Better Eyesight Without Glasses* (New York, NY: Henry Holt & Company, Owl Books, 1981, revised edition).

Chapter 10

33. Henry David Thoreau, "Where I Lived and What I Lived For," *Walden; or, Life in the Woods* (orig. pub. 1854).

Resources

Books

Nature of Reality

Itzhak Bentov, *Stalking the Wild Pendulum: On the Mechanics of Consciousness*. Rochester, VT: Inner Traditions International, Destiny Books, 1988 (reprint edition).

Jane Roberts—All books (the two listed below are good choices for those new to her work).

Jane Roberts and Robert F. Butts (Contributor), *Seth Speaks: The Eternal Validity of the Soul*. San Rafael, CA: Amber-Allen Publishing, 1994 (reissue edition).

Jane Roberts and Robert F. Butts (Contributor), *The Nature of Personal Reality: Specific, Practical Techniques for Solving Everyday Problems and Enriching the Life You Know (A Seth Book)*. San Rafael, CA: Amber-Allen Publishing, 1994 (reissue edition).

Michael Talbot, *The Holographic Universe*. New York, NY: HarperCollins Publishers, HarperPerennial, 1991.

David Tate, *The Shift: A Time of Change (Elias Book One)*. London, United Kingdom: Contact Publishing, 2004.

Fred Alan Wolf, Ph.D., *Taking the Quantum Leap: The New Physics for Non-Scientists*. New York, NY: Harper & Row Publishers, Perennial Library, 1989 (revised edition).

Personal Growth

J. Allen Boone, *Kinship With All Life: Simple, Challenging, Real-Life Experiences Showing How Animals Communicate With Each Other and With People Who*

Understand Them. San Francisco, CA: HarperCollins, HarperSanFrancisco, 1976.

David Cates, *Unconditional Money: A Magical Journey into the Heart of Abundance.* Willamina, OR: Buffalo Press, 1995.

Deepak Chopra, M.D., *Ageless Body, Timeless Mind: The Quantum Alternative to Growing Old.* New York, NY: Random House, Harmony Books, 1994 (reissue edition).

Deepak Chopra, M.D., *The Seven Spiritual Laws of Success.* San Rafael, CA: Amber-Allen Publishing, 1995.

Byron Katie with Stephen Mitchell, *Loving What Is: Four Questions That Can Change Your Life.* New York, NY: Random House, Three Rivers Press, 2003.

Karen Kingston, *Clear Your Clutter With Feng Shui.* New York, NY: Random House, Broadway Books, 1999.

Dr. Eric Pearl, *The Reconnection: Heal Others, Heal Yourself.* Carlsbad, CA: Hay House, 2003.

Elaine St. James, *Simplify Your Life: 100 Ways to Slow Down and Enjoy the Things that Really Matter.* New York, NY: Hyperion, 1994.

Elaine St. James, *Living the Simple Life: A Guide to Scaling Down and Enjoying More.* New York, NY: Hyperion, 1998 (reprint edition).

Personal Care

William H. Bates, M.D., *The Bates Method for Better Eyesight Without Glasses.* New York, NY: Henry Holt & Company, Owl Books, 1981 (revised edition).

Mildred Carter and Tammy Weber, *Body Reflexology: Healing at Your Fingertips.* Paramus, NJ: Parker Publishing Company, Reward Books, 1994 (revised and updated edition).

Louise L. Hay, *Heal Your Body: The Mental Causes for Physical Illness and the Metaphysical Way to Overcome Them.* Carlsbad, CA: Hay House, 2003 (reissue edition).

Peter Kelder, *Ancient Secret of the Fountain of Youth: Book 1*. Gig Harbor, WA: Harbor Press, 1998 (reissue edition).

Christopher S. Kilham, *The Five Tibetans: Five Dynamic Exercises for Health, Energy, and Personal Power*. Rochester, VT: Inner Traditions International, Healing Arts Press, 1994.

Michael Sky, *Breathing: Expanding Your Power and Energy*. Santa Fe, NM: Bear & Company Publishing, 1990.

Websites

Nature of Reality

Biology of Belief (Bruce Lipton, Ph.D.)— *www.brucelipton.com*

Elias Forum—*www.eliasforum.org*

Spirit 2000—*www.spirit2000.com*

Personal Growth

Emotional Freedom Techniques—*www.emofree.com*

PSYCH-K—*www.psych-k.com*

The Work of Byron Katie—*www.thework.org*

For additional recommended books, websites, nutritional products, and personal care products, refer to the Transcend Aging website at *www.transcendaging.com*.

Glossary

Acupressure—Applying pressure to specific points (commonly called **acupressure points**) on the surface of the body to increase energy, alleviate pain, and restore the body to optimal functioning; also see **reflexology**.

Acupressure Points—Precise locations on the body where energy is concentrated; the Chinese mapped these points over a 2,000-year period; also known as **acupuncture points**.

Acupuncture—A traditional Chinese medical practice in which health problems are treated by inserting fine needles into the body at precise points.

Acupuncture Meridians—A network of energy channels throughout the body, on which various **acupuncture points** are located.

Acupuncture Points—Precise locations on the body where energy is concentrated; the Chinese mapped these points over a 2,000-year period; also known as **acupressure points**.

Anabolism—Synthesis; rebuild and repair processes.

Anthocyanins—**Flavonoids** in plant pigments ranging from blue to violet to red; biologically active compounds that are powerful antioxidants with numerous health benefits.

Antioxidant—a substance that protects body cells from the damaging effects of oxidation, which is caused by **free radicals**.

Ayurveda (pronounced "eye-ur-vay-dah")—*Ayur* means *life* and *veda* means *science* in Sanskrit; an ancient Indian system of holistic health.

Bates Method—Developed by Dr. William H. Bates; techniques for improving eyesight that help eliminate the need for corrective lenses in many individuals.

Carnivore—An animal that eats mostly flesh foods.

Carotenoids—Plant pigments ranging from yellow to orange to red; biologically active compounds that are powerful antioxidants with numerous health benefits.

Catabolism—Breakdown; wear-down and teardown processes.

Chakra—Means *wheel* in Sanskrit; one of the nonphysical energy centers associated with the physical body.

Cortisol—The major adrenal cortex hormone; it is active in protein and carbohydrate metabolism and is released in greater quantities in response to stress.

Dehydroepiandosterone (DHEA)—A steroid hormone produced by the adrenal glands that can be converted to other steroid hormones; it is believed to counteract some of the biological effects of age-related degeneration.

Dental Fluorosis—Irregular calcification, mottling, weakness, and discoloration of teeth; a permanent condition caused by overexposure to fluoride while the teeth are developing.

Dermis—The lower, connective tissue layer of the skin that contains nerve endings, oil and sweat glands, and blood and lymph vessels.

Dissociative Identity Disorder (DID)—A mental condition in which a person has distinct subpersonalities that are not all aware of one another; formerly known as Multiple Personality Disorder.

Effectors—Cellular proteins that carry out cell behavior.

Ellagic Acid—A phenolic compound with antibacterial, antiviral, and anticancer properties; present in high concentrations in red raspberries, strawberries, and walnuts.

Emotional Freedom Techniques (EFT)—Developed by Gary H. Craig; an energy psychology therapy that is a form of Thought Field Therapy, which treats emotional problems by correcting energy field disruptions by tapping on **acupressure points** while the person being worked on "tunes in" to his or her problem.

Energy Healing—Restoring to a state of balance (health) by means that affect the body's nonphysical energy centers and energy field.

Energy Psychology—A collective description of the various therapies for addressing emotional issues based upon the premise that emotional (and some physical) problems are characterized by disruptions in the body's energy field, and that these problems can be treated with methods that affect the energy field.

Enucleated—With the nucleus removed.

Epidermis—The outer, protective layer of the skin.

Exfoliate—To remove a layer of flakes or scales, such as from the skin.

Facial Tapping—A technique for stimulating **acupressure points** and improving circulation to the face; performed by using the fingertips to tap briskly all over the face and head.

Feng Shui (pronounced "fung shway")—*Feng* means *wind* and *shui* means *water* in Chinese; the Chinese art of placement, used for interior and exterior design.

Five Tibetans (also known as the **Tibetan Rites of Rejuvenation**)—Believed to have originated in Tibet; a yoga-like exercise routine said to prevent aging by activating the body's nonphysical energy centers; consists of five basic rites plus an optional sixth rite.

Flavonoids—Plant chemicals that are potent antioxidants with antiviral and antibacterial properties and numerous health benefits; includes the **anthocyanin** group.

Free Radical—One or more atoms that have at least one unpaired electron; in the body, an oxygen molecule that has lost an electron and stabilizes itself by taking an electron from a nearby molecule, resulting in cell damage.

Genetically Engineered Foods—In these foods, a segment of the genetic code has been modified to enhance specific traits such as growth rate, appearance, flavor, shelf life, or resistance to disease or pests.

Genetically Modified Organisms (GMOs)—Contained in **genetically engineered foods**, these may be microorganisms that act as biopesticides or seeds that have been altered genetically to improve a plant's growth rate, appearance, flavor, shelf life, or resistance to disease or pests.

Global Characteristics—Patterns expressed in many diverse aspects of a person's life; examples include perfectionism, impulsiveness, procrastination, overindulgence, thoroughness, and neatness.

Glycemic Index—Related to the rise in blood glucose that results from eating a carbohydrate food.

Hatha Yoga (pronounced "hat-ha yoga")—The branch of **yoga** that involves the practice of physical postures; also see **yoga**.

Herbivore—An animal that eats mostly plant foods.

Holistic—Emphasizing the importance of the whole and the interdependence of its parts; the term is used to describe more natural alternatives to conventional medical therapies.

Integral Membrane Proteins (IMPs)—Special cellular proteins; **receptors** and **effectors**.

Lutein—A plant chemical in the **carotenoid** family that is particularly beneficial for the eyes; present in high concentrations in bilberries, kale, spinach, and other dark green leafy vegetables.

Lycopene—A plant chemical in the **carotenoid** family that is beneficial for the vascular system and has anticancer effects (particularly for prostate cancer); present in high concentrations in red vegetables and fruits.

Mahasamadhi—The Sanskrit term for a yoga master's final exit from the physical body.

Mantra—A word or phrase repeated in meditation, prayer, or incantation.

Micronized—Ground into tiny particles, as is done to the zinc oxide and titanium dioxide used in modern sunscreens.

Mindfulness—Incorporating meditation into daily life by paying attention to what you are doing in the moment, without having extraneous thoughts.

Molecular Distillation—A purification process in which a substance is heated under vacuum with such low pressure that no intermolecular collisions can occur before condensation.

Observer Effect—The influence of a conscious observer on matter and energy.

Organelle—A structure within a cell that performs a differentiated function.

Palming—An eye relaxation technique performed by cupping the hands over closed eyes to block out as much light as possible.

Paradigm—A set of assumptions, concepts, values, and practices that constitutes a way of viewing reality.

Phospholipids—The major structural lipids (fats) of most cellular membranes.

Probiotics—Beneficial bacteria (such as *L. acidophilus*, *B. bifidus*, and *L. reuteri*) that normally populate the intestines and are necessary for proper digestion.

Psychoneuroimmunology—A field of study that explores how the mind affects the body, including its effects on the immune, endocrine, nervous, cardiovascular, and digestive systems.

PSYCH-K—Developed by Robert M. Williams, M.A.; an energy psychology therapy that works by increasing communication between the two brain hemispheres and facilitating direct communication with the subconscious mind, enabling people to alter their beliefs and maximize their potential.

Quantum—Something that can be measured; a discrete quantity or amount.

Quantum Physics—The branch of physics that uses **quantum theory** to describe and predict the qualities of a physical system.

Quantum Theory—A theory in physics based on the principle that matter and energy have the properties of both particles and waves.

Qi Gong (pronounced "chee gong" or "chee kung")—*Qi* means *breath of life* or *life force* and *gong* means *mental control of the body* in Chinese; an ancient Chinese discipline that stimulates the flow of life force energy by using controlled breathing and movements.

Receptors—Cellular proteins that act as the "sense organs" of the cells.

Reflexology—A practice that involves applying pressure to specific points (commonly called **acupressure points**) on the surface of the body to increase energy, alleviate pain, and restore the body to optimal functioning; the term is most often used to refer specifically to pressure applied to the feet and hands; also see **acupressure**.

Tapotement—A massage technique that involves using the fingertips to lightly tap areas of the face or body.

Therapeutic Touch—Developed in the early 1970s by Dolores Krieger, Ph.D., R.N. with her mentor Dora Kunz; a method of energy therapy derived from the ancient practice of laying-on-of hands; used extensively by nurses and other health practitioners worldwide.

Thought Field Therapy (TFT)—Developed by Roger J. Callahan, Ph.D.; an energy psychology therapy that treats emotional problems by correcting energy field disruptions by tapping on **acupressure points** while the person being worked on "tunes in" to his or her problem.

Tibetan Rites of Rejuvenation (also known as the **Five Tibetans**)—Believed to have originated in Tibet; a yoga-like exercise routine said to prevent aging by activating the body's nonphysical energy centers; consists of five basic rites plus an optional sixth rite.

Toning—Using the human voice to release tensions and restore the body to a balanced, healthy state.

Triple-A Process—A three-step method for dealing with negative feelings about something; the steps are Acknowledge, Address, and Abandon.

Vegan—A diet that excludes all animal products (meat, fowl, fish, dairy, eggs, and honey).

Vegetarian—A diet that includes plant food and animal products such as dairy and eggs, but no flesh foods (meat, fowl, or fish).

Victim Mentality—The belief that you have no choice; the belief that something can be foisted upon you by another person or an outside force.

Yoga—Means *union* in Sanskrit; an ancient Indian art based on a harmonizing system of development for the mind, body, and spirit.

Zeaxanthin—A plant chemical in the **carotenoid** family that is particularly beneficial for the eyes; present in high concentrations in kale, spinach, and other dark green leafy vegetables.

Index

A

Acupressure 67, 82, 112, 113, 116, 147, 149, 152
Acupressure points 67, 112, 147, 149, 152
Acupuncture 76, 78, 81, 82, 147
Acupuncture meridians 147
Acupuncture points 82, 147
Adrenal 35, 106, 148
Anabolism 14, 15, 147
Anthocyanins 92, 147
Antioxidant 147
Ashwagandha 95
Aspartame 93
Ayurveda 147

B

Bates Method 117, 141, 144, 147
Bates, William H. 117, 141, 144, 147
Bhringaraj 95
Biology of Belief 13, 139, 145
Birch Trees 115
Birthdays 23, 26
Breathing 12, 36, 37, 66, 102, 103, 104, 105, 106, 140, 145, 152

C

Callahan, Roger J. 67, 152
Carnivore 89, 148
Carotenoids 91, 92, 148
Carter, Mildred 83, 141, 144
Catabolism 14, 148
Chakra 105, 148
Chlorophyll 92

Clutter 51, 124, 127, 144
Conscious creation 41, 50, 58
Cortisol 35, 148
Cosmetic 8, 9, 20, 21, 23, 61, 118, 119
Craig, Gary H. 148

D

Death 3, 13, 49, 90, 129, 130, 131, 132, 133, 134
Decluttering 125, 127
Dehydroepiandosterone (DHEA) 35, 148
Dental 9, 89, 116, 117, 148
Dental fluorosis 116, 148
Dermis 114, 148
Dissociative Identity Disorder (DID) 21, 148
Drugs, over-the-counter 84, 85
Drugs, pharmaceutical 7, 8, 67, 77, 84, 95

E

Eclipta alba 95
Effector 14
Elias ix, 105, 106, 108, 140, 141, 143, 145
Ellagic acid 92, 148
Emotional Freedom Techniques (EFT) 67, 148
Energy center ix, 81, 102, 105, 106, 107, 108, 109, 110, 141, 148, 149, 152
Energy healing 1, 79, 81, 82, 130, 149
Energy psychology 66, 67, 68, 69, 148, 149, 151, 152
Ennis, Mary ix, 105, 140
Enucleated 13, 149
Epidermis 114, 149
Essential Fatty Acid (EFA) 93

Exercise 2, 8, 9, 11, 13, 18, 36, 37, 38, 55, 60, 81, 96, 99, 100, 103, 149, 152
Exfoliate 112, 149

F
Facial tapping 112, 113, 149
Feng shui 59, 144, 149
Five Tibetans 102, 103, 109, 141, 145, 149, 152
Flavonoids 91, 92, 147, 149
Flaxseed 92
Fluoride 85, 97, 116, 117, 148

G
Genetically engineered foods 90, 91, 150
Genetically Modified Organisms (GMO) 90, 150
Global characteristics 39, 150
Glycemic index 94, 150
Gynostemma 95

H
Hair 7, 16, 43, 53, 54, 55, 56, 58, 61, 62, 63, 85, 93, 95, 111, 116
Hay, Louise L. 80, 140, 144
He shou wu 95
Hemp 93
Hempseed oil 93
Herb 95, 96
Herbal 36, 95, 112
Herbivore 89, 150
Holistic 75, 76, 77, 78, 79, 82, 147, 150
Honey 94, 153
Horsetail 95

I
Integral Membrane Protein (IMP) 14, 150
Intuition 1, 32, 33, 34, 82, 107, 118

K
Kelder, Peter 102, 103, 141, 145
Kilham, Christopher S. 103, 141, 145

L
Liberman, Jacob 141
Lipton, Bruce H. 13, 139
Longevity 88, 95, 129
Lutein 92, 118, 150
Lycopene 92, 150

M
Mahasamadhi 130, 150
Mantra 34, 150
Martin, Stephen Hawley 16, 139
Meditation 34, 35, 36, 37, 106, 140, 150, 151
Micronized 114, 115, 151
Mindfulness 34, 151
Molecular distillation 93, 151
Money 8, 48, 49, 51, 52, 77, 97, 98, 100, 111, 124, 128, 144

N
Nail buffing 116
Nutiva 93
Nutrition 1, 2, 87, 94, 97, 112
Nutritional supplements 7, 8, 9, 20, 77, 94, 123

O
Observer effect 151
Organelle 14, 151
Organic 85, 90, 91, 93

P
Palming 117, 118, 151
Paradigm 2, 5, 10, 22, 77, 151
Pert, Candace 1
Phospholipid 14, 151
Plastic surgery 8, 23, 118, 119

Probiotic 85
Procrastination 38, 39, 150
PSYCH-K 68, 145, 151
Psychoneuroimmunology 1, 151

Q
Qi gong 102, 152
Quantum 73, 139, 143, 144, 151, 152
Quantum physics 73, 151
Quantum theory 151, 152

R
Ragnar, Peter 22, 140
Receptor 14
Reflexology 82, 83, 113, 141, 144, 147, 152
Roberts, Jane ix, 41, 45, 140, 143

S
Self-acceptance 57
Shavegrass 95
Skin 7, 8, 21, 53, 74, 85, 93, 94, 95, 106, 111, 112, 113, 114, 115, 116, 148, 149
Sky, Michael 37, 140, 145
Stevia 94
Sun 113, 114, 115, 116
Sunglasses 114
Sunscreen 112, 114, 115, 116
Sweeteners 93, 94

T
Talbot, Michael 83, 139, 143
Tapotement 112, 152
Teeth 84, 89, 95, 96, 106, 113, 116, 117, 148

Therapeutic Touch 82, 152
Thoreau, Henry David 123, 142
Thought Field Therapy (TFT) 152
Tibetan Rites of Rejuvenation 102, 103, 149, 152
Titanium dioxide 115, 151
Tobacco 84
Toning 107, 108, 109, 152
Triphala 96
Triple-A process 60, 152

V
Vegan 153
Vegetarian 153
Victim mentality 63, 64, 73, 153
Vision 21, 92, 95, 104, 117, 118
Visualization 55, 56, 107, 108, 109, 110

W
Water 11, 13, 36, 39, 48, 52, 60, 64, 80, 83, 85, 91, 96, 97, 111, 116, 117, 149
Weber, Tammy 83, 141, 144
Weight 7, 55, 57, 62, 88, 93, 96, 97, 98, 100, 105, 124
Williams, Robert M. 17, 68, 139, 151
Winter cherry 95
Wolf, Fred Alan 139, 143

Y
Yoga 23, 100, 101, 102, 130, 149, 150, 152, 153

Z
Zinc oxide 114, 115, 151

0-595-31812-6

Printed in the United States
127379LV00005B/11/A